Praise for
Conquering Postpartum Depression

"The only word I could think of when reading this book was 'life-saver.' Women and their families will feel not only comforted by the up-to-date and practical information, but will feel that their lives will be saved by the knowledge that their symptoms can be so easily and successfully treated."

> —Alice Domar, Ph.D., author of *Healing Mind,*
> *Healthy Woman* and *Self Nurture: Learning to Care*
> *for Yourself as Effectively as You Care for Everyone Else*

"This is certainly a book that will be on my bookshelf, and I will strongly recommend it as reading to any patient and her family dealing with postpartum depression. In this era of HMO medicine, few physicians devote the time needed to explain all the issues involved with this all-too widespread problem. This excellent book provides the extensive consultation that these women need."

> —Mary Jane Minkin, M.D.

"This is a thoughtful, comprehensive, and user-friendly guide. Women struggling with postnatal mood disorders will identify with the case histories and find hope for their own recovery in the stories."

> —Anne Buist, MD, Director of the Australian
> National Postnatal Depression Program

"Babies need happy mothers. This book will help this happen."

> —William Sears M.D., co-author of *The Baby Book*

Conquering
Postpartum
Depression

A PROVEN PLAN FOR RECOVERY

Ronald Rosenberg, M.D.

Deborah Greening, Ph.D.

James Windell, M.A.

Da Capo
LIFE
LONG

A Member of the Perseus Books Group

Many of the designations used by manufacturers and sellers to distinguish their products are claimed as trademarks. Where those designations appear in this book, and where Da Capo Press was aware of a trademark claim, the designations have been printed in initial capital letters.

Text design by Brent Wilcox
Set in 11-point Simoncini Garamond by The Perseus Books Group

Cataloging-in-Publication data for this book is available from the Library of Congress.

First Da Capo Press paperback edition 2004
ISBN 0-7382-0951-1

Published by Da Capo Press
A Member of The Perseus Books Group
http://www.dacapopress.com

Da Capo Press books are available at special discounts for bulk purchases in the U.S. by corporations, institutions, and other organizations. For more information, please contact the Special Markets Department at the Perseus Books Group, 11 Cambridge Center, Cambridge, MA 02142, or call (800) 255–1514 or (617) 252–5298, or email special.markets@perseusbooks.com.

1 2 3 4 5 6 7 8 9—08 07 06 05 04

Contents

CONTENTS

Acknowledgments

No book is a product of the authors alone. This is certainly true of this book as there are a number of people who assisted us, both directly and indirectly.

We would like to thank Dr. Alan Rosenbaum for his longtime commitment to women's health care, and kindness in mentoring us and providing a comprehensive treatment environment that gave us a start. Furthermore, Dr. Rosenbaum deserves special recognition because he has been instrumental in bringing the psychopharmacological treatment of women to the forefront in metropolitan Detroit.

Dr. Lee Cohen, director of reproductive psychiatry at Massachusetts General Hospital, has been a source of inspiration because of his excellence in providing care and research in postpartum depression.

The American College of Obstetricians and Gynecologists also deserves thanks for their dedication to the health care of women.

Marie Osmond deserves a standing ovation for bringing her own story of postpartum depression to the awareness of countless women who needed someone to speak out and describe what it feels like to live through postpartum depression.

There are a number of people who generously provided us support and their own personal stories throughout the writing of this book. In particular we would like to thank Karen Schroeder; the staff at the Beaumont Hospital Parenting Center in Royal Oak, Michigan, which includes Beth Fryblewicz, Deanna Robb, and Julie Kouziak; and Vickie

Rupert, Katie Conti, and Deb Farwell. We want to thank many other people whom we could never begin to name. However, these women and their husbands were open and honest in sharing aspects of their personal life—all with the intention of helping other women and families. The women who allowed us to use their quotes and their often painful personal situations in the writing of this book deserve our special gratitude.

We want to thank the many obstetricians and gynecologists in the Detroit area who are compassionate, caring, and willing to listen to their patients and to send those patients for treatment. And we want to thank all of those people in the health care community for their receptivity to our team approach to treating postpartum depression.

Finally, we want to thank our agent, Denise Marcil, who believed in this book from the beginning, and to our editor, Marnie Cochran, who was the intellectual midwife who has helped to shape it into the story we wanted to tell.

Authors' Note

It's often difficult to determine how it is that people with diverse backgrounds come together to work as a team with a common cause. We're not exactly sure why our paths were destined to cross and how it was that we ended up in the same place, but that's exactly what happened. And we're not just talking about our work with postpartum depression—all three of us authors, remarkably, live in the same neighborhood.

It might be destiny, but the fact is we each took different roads in order to end up together helping women and their families overcome postpartum depression (PPD). For example, Ron Rosenberg remembers exactly what case represented a turning point in his professional life when he was practicing as an obstetrician and gynecologist. The day after Ron delivered Samantha's baby, he stopped in her hospital room to see how she was doing. Samantha was not doing well at all. She was severely depressed and talking in a way that frightened Ron. He immediately transferred her to the psychiatric ward of the hospital—a move that was not only extremely unusual at the time, but highly criticized. There she was treated with medication and within a few days was able to go home and care for her baby.

Three years later, Samantha's husband made an appointment at Ron's office to talk. He said he came to thank him for saving the lives of both his wife and his child. It was that thank you from a husband and father that galvanized a thought that had been circling in Ron's head for a few years into a plan of action. He would return to a second residency and become a psychiatrist.

"I knew that as a psychiatrist I could do more for depressed mothers than I could as an obstetrician," Ron says. "They needed someone to listen to them and take their emotional needs seriously."

Debby Greening, after raising three daughters, went back to graduate school to get a Ph.D. in psychology. She began working with women who had been traumatized. "I was really drawn to these women who had been through so much," Debby says now. "Maybe that was because of the trauma I had experienced in my own life, especially during pregnancy, that I felt like I wanted to help other women."

Working through the court system, she was counseling traumatized women who had been assaulted or victimized by a violent husband or partner. Finally out of school, she was excited, enthusiastic, and passionate about her work. Over time, she found herself frequently frustrated that she wasn't helping as many women as she thought she could—or as much as she had hoped. "The cognitive behavioral psychotherapy I was practicing," Debby says, "wasn't helping many of these women who were so anxious and depressed that they often couldn't even leave their homes to come to my office for treatment."

Over time, she learned that many of her colleagues were referring their clients to a psychopharmacologist who specialized in women who were difficult to treat because of a serious depressive or anxiety disorder. "I began to hear the name Ron Rosenberg," Debby remembers, "and what I kept hearing was that Dr. Rosenberg often seemed to work miracles with his use of medication."

Soon, she began making referrals to Dr. Rosenberg, and he began referring women to her for individual or group therapy. Planned or not, Debby Greening was beginning to treat—and even to specialize in treating—women with mood disorders, including postpartum depression.

During an internship while completing her Ph.D., Debby worked at a juvenile court psychological clinic, where James Windell was on the staff. Jim, the author of several parenting books, had developed a parent training program for parents of delinquents. During Debby's year-long internship, she and Jim became friends, although it would be a few years before they started working together. In the meantime, she continued to work in the court system as well as in women's shelters where she counseled thousands of people involved in violent relationships. She would also work with judges and referees in the courts in the role of expert witness and consultant, which led to certification in forensic medicine and as a forensic examiner.

As Debby continued to treat women, she began to realize that there was a major ingredient missing in her attempts to aid the healing of women. That missing ingredient was the role of parenting. "The women I was working with were frightened of their own babies," Debby has said. "They were terrified of not being good enough mothers, they were terrified of not meeting their own expectations, and ultimately, they were terrified of failing completely. Many of these women had only one road map to follow—that of their own mothers—and that was often not the map they wanted. And that frightened them even more. But I didn't always know how to help them either."

That's where Jim came in. While he was working with delinquent and defiant children and adolescents, both in and out of the juvenile court system, he had come to believe that many of these kids had spent the first few years of their lives with one or more depressed parents. Often the depressed parent was the mother. When Debby related her work with women with postpartum depression and asked him to become part of the emerging "postpartum team," he began to see that postpartum depression could be the link that helped him make sense of the problems that children developed in school and in the community.

The Postpartum Depression Team

Together we bring to the table more than sixty-five years of experience working with women and families. More importantly, our efforts to help women with postpartum depression have enabled us to develop a treatment program that has been proven to be effective. Because each of us brings something different to this working relationship, we now see the team approach as essential in the successful treatment of postpartum depression.

Besides being an obstetrician/gynecologist, a psychiatrist, a psychopharmacologist, and an addictionologist, Ron Rosenberg is one of only a few doctors in the United States who has practiced the two specialties of OB/GYN and psychiatry simultaneously. Prior to becoming a doctor, Ron studied pharmacology at the University of Michigan. As an obstetrician and gynecologist he has been chief resident at William Beaumont Hospital in Royal Oak, Michigan, one of the largest hospitals in the country. He has also been in charge of the Obstetrics and Gynecology Department at William Beaumont Hospital in Troy, Michigan. These credentials and experiences make him especially skilled in treating women with mood disorders and with treatment-resistant depression. Ron is dedicated to helping women who have "fallen through the cracks" and have suffered longer and more severely than necessary.

Debby Greening's work as a clinical psychologist in private practice, as well as a consultant and expert witness in the area of domestic violence, stalking, and family violence, gives her special insight into the psychological stress experienced by women. In her private practice over the last several years, she has conducted group and individual therapy sessions with hundreds of women suffering from postpartum depression. She has arguably had more experience with women's postpartum depression groups than any other psychologist.

Jim Windell published his first parenting book, *Discipline: A Sourcebook of 50 Failsafe Techniques for Parents,* in 1991. Since then he has written seven books, all devoted to helping parents with various issues in the struggle to raise healthy children. As an author, court psychologist, and newspaper columnist, his focus has been on teaching parents for much of his career.

"Raising children is one of the hardest jobs in the world," he says. "However, these days the job seems to be compounded by numerous new and unique stressors. In addition, we know more about what is involved in raising well-adjusted children. The mental health of the mother in the early months and years of life is critical."

It is because of this concern that we teamed up to bring together the skills he's developed in helping parents be more effective. Each of us brings a unique background and expertise to the team. And that, we feel, is essential in helping depressed women.

Introduction

Like girls almost everywhere, Lisa grew up playing with dolls. She never seemed to tire of feeding, changing, bathing, and dressing her babies. Lisa took them for long walks and summer picnics. She had entire conversations with her dolls, pretending that they were all part of her family.

Lisa loved playing at being a mommy, and eventually playing house became her favorite pastime with the boys and girls in her neighborhood. They each took on roles, which not surprisingly resembled both the jobs and personalities of their own families. Some kids got to be the children, while others got to be the dad—who drove his car into the driveway when it was time for dinner. Whoever was low on the totem pole had to be the family dog. But Lisa always got to be the mommy. She insisted.

As soon as she was old enough, Lisa began baby-sitting. Earning spending money was a secondary reward, as Lisa was a natural with little ones, truly enjoying their company. By the time her older brothers and sisters had children, Lisa was the one they called to baby-sit. Her siblings even looked to her to reassure them in their new roles as parents. For Lisa, the step to motherhood would be easy and natural. After all, she had been preparing for this all of her life.

After falling in love and getting married to Jason, Lisa's dream came true. She was pregnant. Both Lisa and Jason were ecstatic about becoming parents. As soon as the doctor confirmed she was pregnant,

Lisa and Jason began planning. They would paint the nursery, buy baby clothes, read books about naming their baby, and sign up for a child-birth preparation class at the local hospital where the blessed event would take place.

A few months later, in the first session of their childbirth classes, they felt a sense of camaraderie with the other couples. They compared notes and smiled at stories of the in-laws arguing over what to name their babies. Somehow, that seemed to be the worst problem that any of them could imagine.

At the end of the first class, all the couples were given a handful of brochures, including one with a few paragraphs on postpartum depression. Lisa and Jason quickly scanned it and set it aside, believing that it had nothing to do with them.

Lisa's dream came true when her beautiful baby arrived. However, having her baby was not everything she had ever imagined. What she had never anticipated was postpartum depression. In fact, there are nearly 400,000 women, like Lisa, in the United States each year who ex-perience depression during or after the births of their babies.[1] A major-ity of women, we now know, experience some sort of mood disorder during their pregnancies.[2]

Like Lisa and Jason, most expectant parents look forward to all of the exciting events surrounding a new baby. Depression, though, is not one of the events that's anticipated. Yet, eight out of ten women will ex-perience some form of alteration in their moods during or following pregnancy.[3]

Despite these odds, which are not well understood by most of us, de-pression is a taboo subject. Most people won't talk about it, and in childbirth classes almost no information about postpartum depression is given. Some childbirth classes cover caesarian sections in detail, yet postpartum depression is more likely to occur than a woman having a C-section delivery.[4] A significant number of women and their families wait until there is a crisis before acknowledging that depression has touched their lives. Part of the problem is that depression is not something that you anticipate. It just sneaks up on you—sometimes with shocking abruptness.

Our purpose in writing this book is to take some of the surprise—and a lot of the fear—out of this mood disorder called postpartum depression. We want you to know that there is every reason to be hopeful and reassured. You should understand that if you, or a woman you know or love, is depressed during or following pregnancy, recovery can take place.

In our work with hundreds of women and their families, we have discovered three key ingredients to a restoration of health. These key ingredients, when carefully considered and followed as we suggest, will help you or your loved one return to a pre-pregnancy level of functioning, and will help maintain good health through subsequent pregnancies. These three essential ingredients can assist you in fulfilling whatever dreams or expectations you have of motherhood and raising a family. The three proven keys to recovery from postpartum depression are:

1. Know your postpartum depression risk factors.
2. Make sure you receive a comprehensive assessment for postpartum depression.
3. Receive a multi-dimensional treatment approach by a team of postpartum depression specialists.

You Don't Have to Feel Hopeless

Most everybody who comes through our door has begun to feel a little hopeless. By the time women come to us, many are in the throes of serious postpartum depression. And they all have similar thoughts and feelings: *My life won't go on; I'll never be able to take care of my baby; I'm afraid something will happen to my baby; I've made a mistake having a child; Nobody in my family understands what I'm going through; There's nobody to tell how I really feel; If I do tell somebody how I feel, they might take my baby away.*

As postpartum depression deepens, it becomes more difficult to ask for help. This may be due to both becoming more frightened and, at the same time, having less and less energy. As a result, you may have postponed asking for help. When you become desperate and finally reach out, you may, unfortunately, receive inadequate help. Inadequate help drives fear and hopelessness. Thus begins a downward spiral. When women do ask for help and don't get it, they frequently give up. But it doesn't have to be this way.

If you are depressed, you can get help. You can get better and you can be the mother, the partner, the wife, and the friend you know you can be. In other words, you can be yourself again.

Today there are great advances and, consequently, there is great hope in the treatment of postpartum depression. Specialists can help you follow through with each of our three key ingredients, one at a time, so that you feel you have a team of supportive experts working with you and for you, giving you hope and reassurance every step of the way.

The Myths of Postpartum Depression

In our research and clinical experience, we have encountered many myths about postpartum depression. One of the reasons for writing this book is to dispel some of the enduring myths we hear.

The first myth we have frequently encountered is that postpartum depression is seen as a problem unrelated to the physical ailments of pregnancy or childbirth. That's why postpartum depression is rarely written about in detail in medical and nursing books, and why it's neglected in medical schools. Most obstetricians and gynecologists know relatively little about postpartum depression, and what they do know may be clouded by other myths.

A second myth we encounter is that there is little difference between the "baby blues" and postpartum depression. Because OB/GYNs receive so little training about postpartum depression, they mistakenly reassure women that what they're feeling after delivery "is just a case of the blues and it will pass." Not knowing how to properly diagnose postpartum depression, they just assume that the symptoms will pass in a few weeks.

When Dr. Rosenberg was in medical school, he never heard about postpartum depression. That didn't change much during either of his residencies. Seldom during his OB/GYN residency did he encounter women with "postpartum depression." The reason for this, he later learned, was because postpartum depression was rarely, if ever, diagnosed. Therefore, he wasn't taught how to recognize it or how to treat it. This is the shame that remains in many hospitals where doctors who become OB/GYNs do their residencies. During pregnancy many women go to the emergency room with various symptoms, including panic attacks. However, they are seen briefly and then released. The reason they aren't admitted is because no one is taking the time to listen to what they are saying. Medical doctors, especially trauma specialists in ERs, are trained to deal with physical emergencies, not depression. If you are in distress, you deserve to be heard. And you deserve not to have your symptoms dismissed.

The third myth we see is that postpartum depression isn't serious unless the woman threatens suicide. This was brought home to us in a significant way recently when Dr. Rosenberg was having lunch with a physician. While discussing one of the physician's patients over lunch, Dr. Rosenberg inquired as to why his patient, a woman who seemed to him to have a severe postpartum depression, hadn't been admitted to the hospital. The physician's answer was brief and sad, and one with which we have become familiar: "She isn't suicidal," the physician answered.

We've found that you don't need to be suicidal to be seriously depressed with postpartum depression. There are many other symptoms of postpartum depression that we will describe in detail in this book that will help you and your doctor recognize if that is what you are experiencing.

A fourth myth is that if you wait long enough, your postpartum depression will simply go away on its own. Obviously, if your doctor thinks you just have a mild case of the baby blues, he or she will also think that these mild symptoms will fade away without treatment. The fact is, though, that there is no guarantee that postpartum depression will go away or disappear without treatment. Many women have suffered for months or years because they thought or were told that their symptoms would pass. What sometimes starts out as a mild case of postpartum depression can develop into a severe, debilitating postpartum depression that can seriously affect you, your baby, and your family.

A fifth myth that is so endemic in our society that it has become "truth" is that postpartum depression can be treated without medications. Psychotherapy can be helpful in treating depression, but most cases of postpartum depression will require one of the effective medications we have available to us these days. You are very likely a woman who dislikes taking pills, or you may believe in treatment with herbs or other alternative methods. Yet we will show you where taking pills may be in your best interest. We will also explain the errors in some alternative treatments that even doctors may engage in when treating postpartum depression.

A sixth myth is that most medications used in the treatment of postpartum depression will have an adverse effect on your baby, and therefore all medications must be avoided while you are breast-feeding. The truth is that many research projects have looked at the question of whether infants are negatively affected when the mother is taking medication. There are, in fact, medications that experts agree are safe. Furthermore, the risks of being depressed and not being adequately treated are generally far greater than the risks of taking medication while being effectively treated and breast-feeding.

Understanding the Three Key Ingredients in the Postpartum Depression Recovery Program

The first of the three key ingredients in an effective program for recovering from postpartum depression is to **know your risk**. If you think about it, it's not any different than knowing your family history for such physical ailments as diabetes or high blood pressure. Exploring and understanding your risk for experiencing postpartum depression will give you a sense of control. You can start planning earlier and decrease your fear.

Pam was diagnosed with PPD only after suffering the agony of a devastating depression several weeks after her first child was born. It was a rough several months before she was fortunate enough to find a psychiatrist who specialized in treating postpartum depression. The psychiatrist prescribed an initial dose of medication and referred Pam to a psychologist for counseling and support.

Three years later, when she got pregnant with her second child, Pam knew she was a prime candidate for a second episode of depression. Having suffered an initial episode, she was realistic about the chances that she would experience the same symptoms again. Pam, therefore, took the important step of making an appointment early in her new pregnancy with the treatment team who had helped both she and her husband through her previous depression.

Since depression runs in families, when Pam's older sister Nancy got married, the two sisters talked about risk factors to developing PPD. Besides family history, Nancy learned that she had at least one other major risk factor—a previous history of depression. She listened to what her sister had to say.

When Nancy eventually became pregnant, they talked again. Nancy asked Pam for the names of the specialists she had seen for PPD. Nancy then made appointments with them and learned she had an additional risk factor she hadn't thought of, that of marital problems. By learning more about her risk for PPD, she could try to decrease her risk while still pregnant. She could also be supported through her pregnancy and after the birth of her baby by the same team of specialists who had helped her sister.

Both Pam and Nancy were prepared to pay attention to the second key ingredient: **getting a comprehensive assessment.** By returning to the psychiatrist with whom she had developed a relationship, Pam was ensuring she would get an appropriate assessment. The psychiatrist could work as part of a team with her obstetrician to monitor her mood throughout the second pregnancy and the months following delivery.

Nancy, too, was in a position to have a comprehensive assessment. The specialist she went to began to assess her mood the day after she gave birth to her son. It was important for the specialist to determine if a history of diabetes in her family would cause her to look depressed and whether there might be a thyroid condition that might also appear as postpartum depression. By ruling out these conditions, her doctor was able to begin to confidently treat her postpartum depression.

Because Pam went to her former therapist early in the pregnancy, she was able to engage in the third key ingredient in the program: **multi-dimensional treatment from a team of specialists.** Pam scheduled visits with her former therapist and returned to her psychiatrist for a medication that had helped ease her depression previously. Together, they discussed Pam's concerns about her depression. Her therapist helped her develop coping skills that would ensure a more positive experience. With encouragement, Pam attended a treatment group with other women going through a similar experience.

Nancy was fortunate in having a treatment team consisting of a psychiatrist, a sensitive obstetrician, helpful nurses, and her therapist. Because of the conflicts in her marriage, Nancy and her husband had counseling with a marital therapist, which helped to increase the presence and support of her husband. She and her husband soon discovered during counseling that they had incompatible views about raising their child. Their therapist recommended a parent skills training class that helped them to learn new techniques and find some common ground for discipline and care for their child.

The treatment plan for Pam also included preparation for her new task of raising both a toddler and an infant—an experience that would be unique for Pam. Being coached and getting expert advice about parenting was critical in the lives of Pam's children. With an expert guiding her, she was able to bond with both children, at the same time providing the stimulation and guidance that each child would need to thrive.

We've learned a number of things over the past several years about treating women with postpartum depression. One of the most important things we've discovered is that all three of these ingredients are essential to a successful treatment program. We've also learned that treatment has to be multi-dimensional or, to put it in medical terms, biopsychosocial. What this means is that treatment cannot include just one approach. Instead, it must consist of psychological counseling with individual and/or group therapy, medication, and social support and parenting advice. If you leave out any part of this treatment, it's like choosing between your biology and your personality. No woman is one-dimensional. Consequently, your treatment must not be, either. You are not just your physical body; nor are you just your mind. You are a social person, a parent, a wife or partner, and perhaps many other things. If all you do is take medication, then this is the same as saying that you are only a bundle of nerves, muscles, and chemicals. If you just get psychotherapy when you also need medication, then this is the same as saying that all you have to do is learn to control your thoughts and emotions. You also may not even be able to concentrate on therapy if your brain chemistry is not regulated. If you have a good support system but that's all you have, then you are being treated as if your interactions with other people are all that you need to feel good. We have found that the women who succeed in treatment pay attention to their brains, their bodies, and their relationships.

Finally, although treatment consisting of medication, psychotherapy, and an increased social network is essential to your recovery, you can't neglect the parent part of you. You are a parent raising a growing, endlessly fascinating, yet dependent child. In other words, you are the sum of your parts and every part of you—including the part that is devoted to parenting—must be treated in order for you to be whole once again.

What You Will Learn from This Book

Just as we've learned a great deal about postpartum depression over the last several years, we want you to learn all you can about this subject, too. That's our main reason for writing this book. Our goal is that the book will help you to be well informed about postpartum depression. While this book is not technical or heavily footnoted, that doesn't mean we don't know the literature and the research on postpartum depression. In fact, we do. We've spent the last few years reading every research article and study we could find. You can be confident that if you read something in this book, then it is backed up by our own research and our own clinical experience, as well as our knowledge of the current research by others.

In Part One of this book (*Know Your Postpartum Depression Risk*), you will learn what postpartum depression is and how it differs from other kinds of depression and mood disorders that fall within the postpartum spectrum. You'll also learn what the risk factors are for postpartum depression and what can help you to predict your likelihood of having this or any of the other common pregnancy or postpartum disorders. Furthermore, you will discover a test you can take to help you determine if you have postpartum depression and whether you require immediate treatment. Finally, Part One will help you learn what other problems can make the diagnosis of postpartum depression even more difficult.

In Part Two (*Make Sure You Get a Comprehensive Assessment for Postpartum Depression*), we will tell you what a comprehensive postpartum depression assessment is and where you can go to get one. We believe that you should be proactive in your own assessment. Also, in this part of the book you will learn about the role of stress in postpartum depression and the various roadblocks that might hinder you from getting the assessment or treatment you need.

Finally, in Part Three (*Receive Multi-dimensional Treatment from a Specialized Postpartum Depression Team*), you will learn everything you need to know to get the various kinds of treatment you need to conquer your postpartum depression. There is a chapter on medication, so you will know not only which medications we believe are the most effective for postpartum depression, but also which medications are new on the market or new in the treatment of postpartum depression. There is also a chapter on complementary alternative medicine, which will review the approaches that women are spending millions of dollars on but may be hiding from their doctors. These approaches will include herbology, light therapy, and many others. There is also a chapter on psychotherapy, including individual, family, and group counseling. Additionally, there are chapters on social support and parenting training, so that you can be sure your child grows up in the healthiest environment possible.

How This Book Can Help

After reading this book, you will see that you have great hope for recovery. You will learn when you should be concerned, when to ask for help, where to get help, and exactly how to use the three key ingredients as a proven plan to help you get the knowledge, assessment, and treatment you need. You will also know when you are not getting the right care, which will empower you to assist in your own recovery.

A good team of postpartum depression specialists will be supportive and will reassure you that you will heal. They will also help you get the sleep you need, get assistance through counseling, build a support system, and bond with your baby despite your depression. And the day will come when you will not regret your decision to have had a baby. At least, we've never worked with a woman when it didn't turn out this way.

By following the unique three key ingredients of our program for coping with postpartum depression outlined in this book, it is likely you will be able to return to your pre-pregnancy level of functioning and to a sense of emotional well-being. It is not unusual for women to report that they feel significantly better with treatment for postpartum depression than they did even before their pregnancies. This is because some women may have been suffering from mild symptoms of depression, which progressed so gradually in their lives that they didn't realize that they were depressed.

Your chances of getting well, however, increase significantly by knowing more about each of the key ingredients and what is required in each step. They are not difficult. By reading this book, you will be informed and proactive. Often that is the first step in recovery.

∽

Judy, a woman who was successful with our postpartum depression recovery program, asked us to pass a message on to women who read this book:

"My hope for women who suffer from postpartum depression is that they will know that there is help out there," she says. "For me, having postpartum depression was a different experience with my second child because I knew how to get the treatment I needed. I truly understand that knowledge is power, and that knowledge is available to every woman."

We can't say it any better. Increase your knowledge, power, and hope by reading on and starting your recovery.

PART ONE

Know Your Postpartum Depression Risk

What Is Postpartum Depression?

- Postpartum depression means different things to different people.
- Most pregnancies in the United States are complicated by mood disturbances for the mother.
- The "baby blues" affects four out of five mothers, and other postpartum mood or anxiety disorders affect an additional 10–17 percent of mothers.
- Postpartum depression can feature depressed mood or anxiety that ranges from feelings of panic to racing thoughts to excessive worry and even obsessions.
- Postpartum psychosis at its worst affects only about one or two in a thousand women.

It is important in both recovery from postpartum depression as well as prevention of the disorder that you be aware about your risk for developing it. And we believe the more you know about this devastating disorder the better prepared you will be to take the steps necessary to effectively follow the key ingredients that will lead to successful treatment. The first thing you need to know is what postpartum depression is.

So, what exactly is postpartum depression? The answer to this question depends on who you ask:

If you ask the media, postpartum depression is a guaranteed headline when a woman goes crazy and kills her baby. This kind of media coverage terrifies women to the point that they are even less apt to come forward and ask for help if they think they might be depressed. Unfortunately, the sensationalism that surrounds a tragedy related to postpartum psychosis sends a message that you're either "normal" or you're psychotic—and that there is no in-between.

If you ask many physicians and other health care professionals, postpartum depression is a short period of the "blues" after the birth of a baby. It is easily dismissed as a normal response to childbirth that will pass on its own.

If you ask many husbands and fathers, postpartum depression is a frightening black shroud that has enveloped their wives or partners—with no promise of their eventual return. Men frequently ask: "When will I get my wife back?"

If you ask the general public, postpartum depression is a shameful condition that must be hidden. The public shows understanding and compassion toward a woman who miscarries or whose baby has a developmental problem. However, anything short of joy after the birth of a healthy child is viewed as a terrible and unforgivable selfishness. How could a woman have a miracle of a healthy baby and not feel grateful?

If you ask the women who are in the midst of postpartum depression, they will say that it is a living nightmare of the illogic. "I know I'm in there somewhere, but I can't find myself," said one mom in the throes of PPD. Another woman in a postpartum depression support group described her depression as "unrelenting sadness." A third said, "It's a painful, cruel experience that should not be called depression. It's more like indescribable fear and disaster."

As you can see, and perhaps as you know only too well, there is considerable disagreement about what postpartum depression is. We see it as a distinct disorder that is unique and requires extended training to diagnose. If you are feeling depressed or anxious during your pregnancy or up to as late as twelve months or more following childbirth, it is possible that this signals an underlying postpartum depression that should be addressed first before any other diagnosis is made.

Postpartum depression most often appears different from any other depressive, anxiety, obsessive-compulsive, bipolar, or posttraumatic stress disorder. That doesn't mean that postpartum depression doesn't have one or more of the characteristics of those individual disorders. However, postpartum depression is a disorder that presents itself as a unique combination or mixture of symptoms from more than one of the traditional disorders listed above. It is also different from all of the other mood disorders (like bipolar depression) in that it is the only one that is a combination of the irregularities of both hormones and other neurotransmitters.

This disorder is not yet fully understood, and the longer we work with postpartum depression, in some ways, the more humbled we feel. When postpartum depression goes undiagnosed, it sometimes masquerades as marital conflict, sexual disorder, a fear of caring for your baby, or even doubts about whether or not you've made a mistake by having a baby.

What we've just described is more of a medical definition. However, postpartum depression to us is:

- Going through months that follow childbirth (if not many months of a pregnancy, too) in a dark fog that crept in unexpectedly, without an invitation.
- Losing your sense of self as a woman and new mother.
- Fearing the black fog will never lift and that you might be this way forever.
- Having terrible thoughts and fears about your baby and being afraid to talk about them.
- Feeling like you've made a mistake in having your baby and desperately wishing you could turn back the clock.

- Living the secret fear that you will lose the love of those around you because you aren't good enough to do what your own mother did—care for your baby.

Women who are seriously afflicted by this disorder agree that it alters your body, your personality, and even your spirit. You may hate the way you feel, and hate having to wear a mask, lest people see what's really inside. "It's just easier to keep the door closed and stay home with no explanation," says Judith, a depressed mother.

The Postpartum Depression Spectrum of Disorders

Whatever you call it or however you may choose to define it, most births in the United States are complicated by a mood disturbance of some kind for the mother.[1] However, it is important for you to be able to distinguish between what is frequently called the "baby blues" and postpartum depression.

Although the American Psychiatric Association's *Diagnostic and Statistical Manual of Mental Disorders, Fourth Edition* (commonly referred to as the *DSM-IV*), does not classify postpartum mood and anxiety disorders the way we do, we think that our classification of mood disturbances will help you to be more aware of the level of depression or anxiety you are experiencing during and following pregnancy. Furthermore, having a brief and poignant reference guide can help you to know more about what you are feeling and when you need help.

We also want you to be cautious in trying to diagnose yourself. Most mothers weather the baby blues pretty well on their own. However, when it comes to postpartum depression, postpartum anxiety, and postpartum psychosis, we urge you to get help from a specialist. None of these disorders should be taken lightly or brushed off.

You may want to hide your symptoms after your baby is born. If you're doing this, it is probably because you fear that your baby will be taken from you. *Remember you cannot be treated appropriately if you are afraid to reveal what you are thinking or feeling.* Most of the women we see have some obsessive fears or other thoughts that frighten them. If you are frightened and distressed by the thoughts and feelings you have, you should be aware that this strongly indicates that you are still sane. It doesn't mean that you can treat the symptoms yourself. We will tell you why you must get treatment in a later chapter.

If, at any time, you go from fearing that something will happen to your baby to feeling like you could actually hurt her, you should not be alone with your child and you must contact an expert in postpartum depression immediately.

Kristy, the mother of a 4-month-old boy, told us when she was asked to describe postpartum depression: "I know I have the dream—a good husband, a beautiful baby, and the white picket fence. It's everything I dreamed about, but I can't enjoy it right now."

Another new mother, Megan, put her own unique spin on her experiences of severe postpartum depression: "I'm a star home run hitter in a championship game. The bases are loaded. I'm up at bat with a chance to win the game. There are 50,000 people cheering for me, and all I want to do is throw the bat away."

The list that follows shows you how we classify the various mood disorders that women experience related to pregnancy and childbirth. Since most women who suffer from postpartum depression become symptomatic prior to childbirth, we are including depression and anxiety disorders during pregnancy as one of the childbirth-related emotional disorders. This list will help you compare your symptoms to those we typically see.

Depression and Anxiety During Pregnancy

Occurs: Anytime during pregnancy.

Symptoms may include but are not limited to:

- Mood swings or feeling depressed
- Anxiety, irritability, agitation, tearfulness
- Problems with sleep
- Excessive nausea and vomiting
- Excessive weight gain or weight loss
- Extreme trauma during pregnancy
- Obsessions or compulsions during pregnancy (repetitive thoughts and behaviors)

Baby Blues

Occurs: Within 48 hours of delivery and resolves within two weeks of delivery.

Symptoms may include but are not limited to:

- Persistent sadness and tearfulness
- Anxiety, irritability, agitation, fatigue
- Problems with sleep
- Difficulty concentrating

These women ask for help and mobilize everyone around them in an effort to get that help.

Postpartum Depression

Occurs: Up to two years after delivery.

Symptoms are more pronounced and may include but not be limited to:

- Debilitating depression, and suicidal ideation or thoughts about death
- Hopelessness of ever feeling like yourself again

- Feelings of inadequacy as a wife and mother and helplessness
- Difficulty sleeping, too much sleeping
- Lack of interest in the baby and/or self
- Low level of daily functioning, including personal grooming
- Isolation and social withdrawal
- Feelings that if you tell anyone about your symptoms, your baby will be taken away
- Severe mood swings, which may include euphoria, agitation, and explosive episodes
- Spacing or zoning out with an inability to focus on a task
- Significant and unintended changes in eating patterns

These women are not asking for help and are unable to mobilize support around them.

Postpartum Obsessive-Compulsive Disorder

Occurs: Up to two years but often within 48 hours of delivery.

Symptoms include those in postpartum depression, and also may include:

- New, significant, and unreasonable fears, such as harming the baby and/or self, being alone with the baby, driving in the car with the baby, the dark, bathing the baby, being around knives or other potentially dangerous instruments
- "Visions/pictures" of being unable to control something bad happening to baby (including Sudden Infant Death Syndrome or SIDS)
- Mental rehearsal of how to respond should something happen to baby's well-being
- Fear of being blamed should something happen to the baby
- Anxiety, including panic attacks, irritability, agitation

- Body preoccupations and phobias
- Obsessions and compulsions about cleanliness, germs, and contamination
- Checking over and over the same things that usually involve safety, like door locks, fetal monitor, baby's breathing
- Preoccupation with death and dying

Postpartum Psychosis

Occurs: Usually occurs while in the hospital and often starts within 48 hours of delivery.

Symptoms could include all of the above, but in addition and most important will include at least some of the following:

- Visual or auditory hallucinations
- Delusions
- Despair or elation
- Extreme anxiety or agitation
- Suicidal or homicidal ideation
- Hopelessness

Requires immediate attention and hospitalization.

Baby Blues

Kari, 28, recently gave birth to her first child, an energetic and rotund baby boy. Kari and her husband both wanted very much to have a child and were pleased when they learned that she was pregnant.

However, after Kari came home from the hospital and began to establish a routine of caring for her son, she was surprised to find herself feeling sad. She knew she should be happy and couldn't understand why she was tearful every day.

If this sounds familiar to you, then you are among a majority of women. You may have a case of the "baby blues," which is the most common and least serious of the postpartum period disturbances. Often called the "maternity blues," postpartum blues may be part of the aftermath of giving birth to a baby. If you have the blues, they will disappear within a couple of weeks. Should the symptoms persist beyond two weeks or worsen at any time, then you are likely to be suffering from a more serious postpartum mood disorder. Remember that upwards of 85 to 90 percent of all new mothers experience some form of mood complication during or following childbirth,[2] so don't be ashamed to share your feelings with your doctor.

Symptoms of the baby blues can include episodes of tearfulness, irritability, moodiness, restlessness, and anxiety—mixed with times of feeling well. The symptoms begin within 48 hours of delivery, worsen by days five to seven, and should resolve themselves by twelve to fourteen days.[3] Postpartum blues go away on their own without treatment, rarely requiring counseling or psychiatric intervention. They are the result of expected hormonal shifts, as a woman's biochemistry begins to return to a pre-pregnancy level. When the symptoms last longer than two weeks or appear severe, it is important to talk to a specialist, since approximately one in five women with the baby blues will go on to develop postpartum depression.[4]

Postpartum Depression

Kathy had what she described as a wonderful pregnancy. She was excited about having her first baby and she enjoyed everything about being pregnant—from growing a belly to shopping for maternity clothes.

However, a few days before her baby was born, Kathy knew something wasn't right. She had planned to work until a week before her delivery date. However, before her official delivery date arrived, she became so emotionally and physically fatigued she could no longer work. In addition, during the final week of her pregnancy, she began to feel very frightened about both the delivery itself and being responsible for another human being.

"I kept thinking it was nervousness about the doctor saying I might have to have a C-section," Kathy recalls, "but I thought once this was past and the baby was here, I'd be all right."

The day the baby came, Kathy's doctor decided a caesarian section was indeed necessary. Kathy was amazingly calm—even a bit detached. "I actually felt indifferent when my husband was holding the baby for the first time," Kathy says, "like the baby didn't really belong to me."

Once she was home, all Kathy wanted was to crawl into bed and hide from her baby, her husband, and her friends. She says she felt like a "total mess" by the second day she was home from the hospital. Within a few days, Kathy had become hysterical. "I actually told my husband that I wanted to give our daughter away so I could have my life back the way it was before." From that point on, Kathy cried almost continuously and felt like she had ruined everyone's life by bringing a baby into the world.

In contrast to Kari, Kathy has postpartum depression—not the baby blues.

Postpartum depression is a more serious disorder that occurs in 10 to 17 percent of all mothers.[5] The effects of this disorder vary in severity. When women with postpartum depression look back at their pregnancies, many of them see that they had symptoms during the pregnancy but didn't notice them. When they delivered, their symptoms worsened and could no longer be ignored. There are women who have wonderful pregnancies and don't have any symptoms of postpartum depression until after they deliver. In fact, some women hide their symptoms for months or, in some cases, up to a year—which makes it more difficult for some doctors to diagnose.

One of the most important differences between baby blues and postpartum depression is that with baby blues you are more likely and willing to want and ask for help; but with postpartum depression, you may be more inclined to isolate yourself and avoid asking for help. With postpartum depression, you may hide what you're going through while at the same time feeling devastated and ashamed. You may also feel like you did something wrong and that you "should" be able to control it. You may not be willing to reach out for help until either you feel desperate or someone in your family insists you get help. You know something is wrong, but you are probably not sure what it is. If you thought you had postpartum depression, chances are you quickly banished that thought.

Postpartum depression is not just one feeling or a few symptoms. It is not specific or easily identified as a disorder. It could be likened to the spectrum of colors in a rainbow except that a rainbow is orderly, inspiring, and awesome. Postpartum depression's rainbow is either one without color at all, or one whose colors range from shades of gray to black.

The spectrum of this mood disorder can range from an acute period of depression to a more prolonged major depression that can be totally debilitating. Your mood may be very low all the time, or it may swing dramatically from the depths of despair to a feeling of elation in a short period of time.

Typical features of postpartum depression include a depressed mood that you just can't shake and that keeps you from experiencing life and the care of your baby or other children in the way you expected. For some women, there is a component of anxiety that ranges from feelings of excessive worry, to racing thoughts, to outright panic. At its worst, the anxiety can include obsessive and unreasonable thoughts, fears, and behaviors. Postpartum depression is a time of urgency, if not emergency.

The clinical definition of postpartum depression, the one given by and to physicians, comes from the *DSM-IV*. There is no specific diagnosis of postpartum depression. But there is something called "Postpartum Onset Specifier."[6] This means that if a Major Depressive episode occurs within four weeks of childbirth, then Postpartum Onset can be added to one of the other mood disorders, such as Major Depressive Disorder, Bipolar I Disorder, or Bipolar II Disorder (for example, Postpartum Onset with Bipolar I Disorder).

The *DSM-IV* goes on to say that women with postpartum Major Depressive episodes often have severe anxiety, panic attacks, spontaneous crying, disinterest in their new infants, and insomnia. In essence, there is no separate mood disorder called Postpartum Depression, according to the *DSM-IV*.

How helpful is this? And how does it help physicians, particularly psychiatrists, in understanding, diagnosing, and treating postpartum depression? The answer is obvious. It is not much help at all. It is, in our view, not only unhelpful, but it is inaccurate, sexist, dismissive, and contemptuous of women. No wonder postpartum depression, more often than not, goes undiagnosed, untreated, or mismanaged.

But in all fairness to the *DSM-IV*, and those diagnostic manuals that have come before and will come after, it is important to understand that there are two essential reasons that this manual exists. First, by giving a name to each identifiable emotional or brain disorder, it helps all health care professionals communicate through a common language. For example, if one health professional uses the term "depression," another health professional knows that a certain number of symptoms are associated with this condition. One must meet certain criteria in order to be diagnosed with depression. These symptoms may include feeling depressed, feeling hopeless, increased or decreased appetite, increased or decreased sleep, and so on. We can understand a great deal just by having words, like depression, with agreed upon definitions.

The second reason we have a diagnostic manual is for insurance purposes. There is a code for each disorder, and insurance companies can decide whether or not a particular diagnosis is covered.

But what happens when professionals do their jobs "by the book" is that you, like so many women who need our help, don't get it. Professionals need to listen much more closely to you and other women so that what you're telling us can be heard. There may not be any other physical or emotional disorder that is misdiagnosed, undiagnosed, or mistreated so often as postpartum depression. Listening more attentively to women may actually revolutionize the diagnosis of postpartum depression, not only for future diagnostic and statistical manuals, but also, and most important, for effective treatment of this disorder.

Postpartum Obsessive-Compulsive Disorder

Heather began to feel sad and anxious before her baby was born. After she gave birth to Joshua, her anxieties worsened, turning to specific fears about her baby. She didn't want anyone but her husband to hold her baby, for fear that their germs would make the baby ill. She insisted that her husband often wash his hands, as she did, until they were almost raw. She began to fear that food was contaminated. She scrubbed her counters, wore gloves when she handled food or the baby's bottles, and was afraid to take the baby out of the house.

You won't find Postpartum Obsessive-Compulsive Disorder in the *DSM-IV*. And even if Postpartum Onset Specifier could be tacked on to Obsessive-Compulsive Disorder (OCD), it is our experience that OCD and Postpartum OCD are truly different. Over 50 percent of the women we see in our practices have something else, what we call Postpartum OCD. We feel strongly that more research and attention need to be paid to this aspect of the postpartum disorders.

Most every new mother will think or worry from time to time about something happening to her baby. What occurs with many new moms, however, is that they will begin to obsess about one or more particular fears, such as Sudden Infant Death Syndrome. These thoughts may increase to the point that you can't rest or get these thoughts out of your mind. You might even see yourself as being physically responsible for harm coming to your baby. This will naturally be terrifying because you have no idea where such thoughts are coming from or how to control them. You know that no matter what you feel, you would never harm your baby.

So why would you be thinking such strange things over and over? What does it mean? And how do you get rid of these frightening thoughts—especially if you are afraid to tell anyone what you're thinking?

Even if you didn't plan to get pregnant, like most women, you will love and care for your baby once he or she arrives. Most new mothers will have concerns for the health and safety of their new babies. When an obsessive component is added to normal concerns, these concerns seem to quickly snowball into something that is out of control. This is particularly true when a new mother is not sleeping well.

Joni's baby spent two days in the Neonatal Intensive Care Unit. There were two incidents of the baby turning blue, when he stopped breathing for one to two minutes. When Joni and her husband brought the baby home, her husband felt safe because the doctors said everything was okay now. Joni, however, couldn't take her eyes off her baby. She listened for every breath, even breathing in concert with her baby. She worried constantly that the baby would stop breathing. She rehearsed what she would do, and she obsessed about how she would give the baby mouth-to-mouth resuscitation and call 911 at the same time. She even feared that if she couldn't manage both tasks, it would be her fault that the baby didn't get the help he needed.

This can become a vicious cycle, where in addition to obsessive thoughts, women may begin ritualistic behaviors such as checking repeatedly on the baby's breathing in order to protect their baby. This is often accompanied by guilt, shame, and increasing depression, along with feelings of inadequacy as a mother.

If you have similar symptoms, it's always better to tell a specialist in postpartum depression so that you can get help. Hiding obsessive thoughts and compulsive behaviors will not help you to get better.

Postpartum Psychosis

Postpartum psychosis is rare, affecting only about one or two out of every thousand women.[7] Generally, mothers with postpartum psychosis are severely impaired and may have paranoia, visual or auditory hallucinations, and delusions that frequently focus on the infant dying or being demonic. The voices they hear often command the woman to hurt herself or her baby.

Roberta became more withdrawn and depressed as her delivery date neared. Just before she went to the hospital, she believed that she and her baby would die during the delivery. The birth of her little girl, however, occurred without complications. When the nurse first brought Emily for Roberta to nurse, Roberta refused to nurse the baby, telling the nurse that the baby wasn't her daughter.

Within three days, Roberta was hearing voices and seeing things that weren't there. She says she woke up after a nap one day and saw the Angel of Death standing at the foot of her bed. "Kill Emily before she kills you," the Angel of Death commanded her. From that point on, Roberta began to think about ways of killing her baby and herself.

When postpartum psychosis occurs, it is frequently preceded by Bipolar Disorder. However, it requires immediate medical attention and hospitalization. This is not a condition for anyone—either the woman herself or her family—to hide.

By now, you probably have a much better idea of what postpartum depression is. You may also be wondering if there is a simple test to tell if you have it.

2

How Do I Know If I Have Postpartum Depression?

POINTS TO PONDER IN THIS CHAPTER

- Postpartum depression most often goes unrecognized.
- There is no *one* test for postpartum depression, but there are screening devices to help you and your doctor make a postpartum depression diagnosis.
- Mood disorders *during* pregnancy are more common than those following pregnancy.
- Perhaps the most important question is one you can ask yourself.

You Know Yourself Better Than Anyone Else Knows You

You know better than anyone when there is something wrong with you. But you, like many mothers, may reject the idea that you have postpartum depression. We have developed, as a result, a very simple test. This could be the first and most important test you give yourself. It's a simple one-question gut-check:

Do I believe something is wrong with me—that I'm not myself? If you've answered this already by thinking to yourself, "Something is wrong," or if you've remarked in your head that "I'm not myself," then it is time to consider the possibility that you may have postpartum depression. Further, since we know that more women develop depression or anxiety *during* pregnancy (this is often referred to as the antenatal or perinatal period) than they do *following* pregnancy (postpartum period), you should keep track of your mood during the nine months of pregnancy and up to eighteen months following. Keeping a journal is a great way to do that—even a sentence or two a day. Another way is to ask someone close to you to tell you if they see your mood changing significantly. Asking your husband or someone else close to you can be tricky because you could be the type of woman who hides feelings so well you could win an Academy Award! This takes exhaustive energy all by itself—and usually means your husband, your partner, or your best friends may not know exactly how you feel.

How Does Postpartum Depression Get Diagnosed?

If you go to your physician, whether an obstetrician, your child's pediatrician, an internist, or family practioner, how does he or she diagnose postpartum depression? Our experience indicates that your physician may underestimate the severity of what you are experiencing. Doctors often refer to any depression subsequent to a birth of a child as "the blues" and something that will quickly pass. Too often, physicians will see your depression as a natural fluctuation of hormones that will right itself soon. While that is sometimes the case, the frequency with which the symptoms *don't* right themselves suggests the need for more attention to be paid them.

Jane, the mother of two children, recalls that the postpartum depression she experienced with her first child, a boy, was a "nightmare." "I gave birth to Dustin," she remembers, "and then I just went to a horrible place. The anxiety became so severe in the hours after he was born that a doctor in the hospital gave me a sedative to help me sleep."

Things did not get better when Jane went home with Dustin. She couldn't eat. She was fearful of being a bad mother. The anxiety got worse and she had panic attacks. "I didn't know why any of this was happening to me," Jane says. "When I kept calling the obstetrician, he told me to go to the emergency room. I did what he told me, but even there, no one mentioned that I might have postpartum depression. I didn't get the help I needed."

When Jane next saw her obstetrician at six weeks, she had lost all her birth weight, cried constantly, and thought about suicide. "He told me it was *just* the 'baby blues' and prescribed a mild tranquilizer for me." Fortunately, when Jane was checking out, the receptionist wrote the name of a doctor who specialized in postpartum depression on a piece of paper and gave it to her.

Rachel, another mom who came to us, said that she was irrational by the time she got home from the hospital with her daughter Amanda. "I refused to eat, I didn't want to take a shower, and I couldn't sleep," she says. "I called my mother and asked her to take Amanda because I couldn't handle her."

Rachel's husband made an appointment for Rachel with their obstetrician after five days. He told Rachel that she looked like she was possessed, and since she was crying most of the time, she needed help. "I told the doctor what was going on," Rachel says, "and she told me to take Tylenol PM and get some sleep." Even in her condition, Rachel thought this advice was ridiculous, but she couldn't say that to the doctor. Rachel was lucky that when she told her husband what happened, he called the family doctor and asked for a referral for a doctor who could help Rachel.

It's these kinds of personal stories that confirm what more enlightened professionals also report. Dr. Diana Dell, assistant professor in the departments of obstetrics and psychiatry at Duke University, has said that postpartum depression is "the most underrecognized, underdiagnosed, and undertreated obstetrical complication in America."[1]

Besides the Gut-Check Test,
Is There a Test for Postpartum Depression?

Unfortunately, there is no single or simple medical test to determine whether you have postpartum depression. However, there are screening devices and questionnaires that can help you. The Edinburgh Postnatal Depression Scale (EPDS) has been developed to assist health care professionals to detect mothers suffering from postpartum depression.[2] Tested and first used at health centers in Livingston and Edinburgh, Scotland, the EPDS consists of just ten short statements. Complete all ten questions by underlining which of the four possible responses is closest to how you've been feeling during the past week. Take this test now and see how you score. Remember to base your answers only on how you've felt recently, not what others might have said about your behavior.

EDINBURGH POSTNATAL DEPRESSION SCALE[3]

1. I have been able to laugh and see the funny side of things.
   A. As much as I always could
   B. Not quite so much now
   C. Definitely not so much now
   D. Not at all
2. I have looked forward with enjoyment to things.
   A. As much as I ever did
   B. Rather less than I used to
   C. Definitely less than I used to
   D. Hardly at all
3. I have blamed myself unnecessarily when things went wrong.
   A. Yes, most of the time
   B. Yes, some of the time
   C. Not very often
   D. No, never

4. I have been anxious or worried for no good reason.
    A. No, not at all
    B. Hardly ever
    C. Yes, sometimes
    D. Yes, very often

5. I have felt scared or panicky for not very good reasons.
    A. Yes, quite a lot
    B. Yes, sometimes
    C. No, not much
    D. No, not at all

6. Things have been getting on top of me.
    A. Yes, most of the time I haven't been able to cope at all
    B. Yes, sometimes I haven't been coping as well as usual
    C. No, most of the time I have coped quite well
    D. No, I have been coping as well as ever

7. I have been so unhappy that I have had difficulty sleeping.
    A. Yes, most of the time
    B. Yes, sometimes
    C. Not very often
    D. No, not at all

8. I have felt sad or miserable.
    A. Yes, most of the time
    B. Yes, quite often
    C. Not very often
    D. No, not at all

9. I have been so unhappy that I have been crying.
    A. Yes, most of the time
    B. Yes, quite often
    C. Only occasionally
    D. No, never

10. The thought of harming myself has occurred to me.
    A. Yes, quite often

B. Sometimes
C. Hardly ever
D. Never

How Did You Score?

Calculate your score in the following way:

- Your total score is calculated by adding together the scores for each of the ten items.
- Calculate your scores as follows:
  1. A=0, B=1, C=2, D=3
  2. A=0, B=1, C=2, D=3
  3. A=3, B=2, C=1, D=0
  4. A=0, B=1, C=2, D=3
  5. A=3, B=2, C=1, D=0
  6. A=3, B=2, C=1, D=0
  7. A=3, B=2, C=1, D=0
  8. A=3, B=2, C=1, D=0
  9. A=3, B=2, C=1, D=0
  10. A=3, B=2, C=1, D=0
- If your score is 10 or greater, there is a high probability that you are experiencing postpartum depression. If your score is below 10, it is likely that you are not currently depressed.[4]

Research has consistently shown that the EPDS is very sensitive to postpartum depression. Scores above 10 indicate women are seven times more likely to be diagnosed with postpartum depression.[5] The combination of a structured interview in which your health care professional asks questions about how you are feeling, together with a screening device like the EPDS, gives you a higher chance that your depression will be diagnosed.[6] If you identify yourself as experiencing postpartum depression, see Chapter 4 for more information about assessment and be sure to read all of the chapters in Part Three to familiarize yourself with treatment options. It's important that you follow each of the three key ingredients in our postpartum depression recovery program so that you do not have to suffer in silence.

3

What Is My Risk
for Postpartum Depression?

POINTS TO PONDER IN THIS CHAPTER

- Biological, psychological, and social factors contribute to your risk for developing postpartum depression.
- The strongest predictor of developing postpartum depression is *biological*: depression or anxiety during pregnancy.
- *Psychological* risk factors include self-criticism, stress related to pregnancy, childbirth, or parenting, and adverse life events.
- *Social* risk factors include a lack of social or emotional support and low educational level.

What You've Learned So Far About Postpartum Depression

Even though this is only Chapter 3, you have already learned a great deal about postpartum depression and the other mood disorders that women experience. You are well aware that depression is only one of the mood disturbances involving chemical imbalances that can occur during or following pregnancy; you've learned that about 10 to 20 percent of mothers suffer from postpartum depression; and you've learned that postpartum depression is the most frequent complication of childbirth.

Because both depression and anxiety are such common occurrences for new mothers, the symptoms and risk factors should be well known to women and their families, doctors and other health professionals, and the general public. Unfortunately, here is something else you've learned: Postpartum depression is one of the most misunderstood, misdiagnosed, and mistreated disorders in both obstetrics and psychiatry.

Annette attended one of our postpartum depression workshops. She sat through our morning-long presentation and then patiently waited to ask us some questions. "I'm moving to another state soon, and my husband and I are planning to get pregnant. I know my mother had bouts of depression and my father drank a lot. I have had a lot of trouble with my mood during my periods and have had times when I struggled with anxiety over the past couple of years. I'm concerned I might be a serious candidate for postpartum depression. What do you think?"

We told Annette we had to agree with her. But we supported her courage in coming to a postpartum depression workshop and confronting the possibility that she could suffer from a mood disturbance during her pregnancy or after giving birth. We also told Annette that having risk factors doesn't absolutely predict she would indeed have postpartum depression. But knowing she was at risk would give her the advantage of taking some measures to prevent or minimize any mood or anxiety disruption she might encounter. You should assess your risk, also.

It is not really known why some women become depressed after childbirth and others do not. One important factor is simply biology. The physical changes that occur during and following pregnancy are tremendous. Women's hormones increase markedly during pregnancy, followed by a rapid fall at delivery. Psychological factors, such as how you feel about yourself, the quality of your relationship with your own mother, and the strength of your coping skills can also contribute to the development of postpartum depression. Social factors, such as too many outside stressors or the lack of support, can also be related to depression.

For the most part, postpartum depression is likely to result from a combination of all of these factors. The best way, then, of assessing your risk factors for developing postpartum depression is to look at the three categories of risk. This is referred to as the *biopsychosocial* model. We will consider these biological, psychological, and social risk factors in turn.

The Biological Risk Factors

1. Depression or anxiety during pregnancy
2. A previous history of depression
3. Family history of psychiatric disorders, including depression
4. Baby blues (sadness that is not resolved within two weeks)
5. Fertility treatments
6. Voluntary termination of a pregnancy or miscarriage
7. Premenstrual Dysphoric Disorder (or severe premenstrual syndrome)
8. Thyroid dysfunction or polycystic ovary disease

The postpartum period is a time of great changes in the body. Levels of the female hormones, such as estrogen and progesterone, drop sharply in the hours after childbirth. These sharp decreases may trigger depression or anxiety, although not nearly enough is known about the impact of pregnancy and childbirth on the course of depression.[1] Yet, it is certain that changes in a woman's body during pregnancy and childbirth mean that this period of time is anything but a time of stability.[2] For many women, this hormonal instability leads to an increased likelihood of both depression and anxiety.[3]

Your moods depend on hormones and neurotransmitters. Very simply, hormones affect other neurotransmitters in the brain. A normal brain functions well when neurotransmitters and hormones are working the way they should. Neurotransmitters are chemical messengers in the brain that tell the cells what to do. In this way, they regulate mood. When hormones disrupt the balance, a mood disorder may result. The most vulnerable times in a woman's life occur during hormonal events. Certainly, pregnancy and childbirth are two of the most critical examples. In fact, mood disturbances may be an inevitable consequence for the majority of pregnant women if you consider the entire spectrum of mood and anxiety disruptions ranging from "baby blues" to the more serious mood disorders.

The strongest predictor of postpartum depression is a depressed mood during pregnancy.[4] Other kinds of mood disorders, including the anxiety disorders, that occur during pregnancy are also predictive of postpartum depression. Similarly, a previous history of depression is a critical factor in determining your risk for postpartum depression.[5] The "kindling theory of the brain" says that every time you have one episode of depression, you are more at risk for further episodes of depression. The fact is that if you have had one previous episode of depression, your chances of another depressive episode increase by 50 percent. However, if you have had two previous episodes, your chances for another one are as much as 70 percent.

Lorie, the mother of 4-month-old Kevin, recalls that she had been depressed since she was 15 years old. "I first went to a therapist when I was in high school and I started to self-medicate with marijuana," Lorie says.

Steve remembers that he was aware when he married Karen that she had been depressed and was seeing a psychologist from the time she was a young adult. "The strange thing, though, was that she had a great pregnancy with no signs of depression," Steve says. "However, when our son was born, her depression returned and it was worse than ever."

One-third of the women who have had postpartum depression in the past will have a recurrence of symptoms after a subsequent delivery. A study reported in 2002 in the *Journal of Clinical Psychiatry* concluded that every one of the women in a research project who had postpartum "episodes" after the births of their first children also had episodes after subsequent pregnancies.[6] In fact, the risk for a recurrence of postpartum depression, especially when there is another delivery within two years, is as high as 50 percent. As many as 60 percent of women with bipolar disorder will relapse after childbirth.

The baby blues, the milder mood disturbance we discussed in Chapter 1, has been associated with postpartum depression, also.[7] A case of the baby blues or maternity blues that does not go away within two weeks, or that persists and worsens, has been found to predict postpartum depression.

Premenstrual Dysphoric Disorder (PMDD) or severe premenstrual syndrome (PMS), which affects as many as 80 percent of women, is also a predictor of postpartum depression.[8]

If you have a family history of any psychiatric disorder, including depression, anxiety, and bipolar disorders, or a family history of severe hormonal imbalance, you are also at risk for postpartum depression. Other risk factors include fertility treatments,[9] voluntarily terminating a pregnancy,[10] and miscarriage.

Finally, if you have a thyroid dysfunction, you have an increased risk for both depression in general and for postpartum depression. And polycystic ovary disease also ups your risk for postpartum depression.[11]

The Psychological Risk Factors

1. Psychological Distress
   A. Self-criticism
   B. Thoughts of death or dying
2. Stress Related to Motherhood
   A. The health of the baby
   B. Childcare stress
   C. Inadequate parenting

3. Adverse Life Events or Prolonged Stress
   A. Childhood abuse
   B. Marital disharmony or dissatisfaction
   C. Unintended pregnancy
   D. Severe stress or posttraumatic stress disorder during pregnancy and childbirth
4. Shortened Hospital Stay

The second category of postpartum depression risk factors includes those that are psychological in nature. That is, the risk or challenge is not in your biology or in genetics or in misfirings of brain chemicals, but with increased stress and poor coping skills that interfere with your healthy adjustment during pregnancy or after childbirth.

Carrie, at age 31, was sure she would never get pregnant. She married Ron "knowing" that since he had had cancer as a child, he would be sterile. Carrie did not want children, and for she and Ron, this was an ideal arrangement.

When Carrie discovered through a home pregnancy test that she was indeed pregnant, she says she spent the weekend "crying my eyes out." She hoped she would miscarry, but she didn't. "Needless to say," Carrie says, "I did not enjoy being pregnant. I resented the fact that I was pregnant, I hated myself for not using birth control, and I resented the baby I was carrying."

Carrie had more than one type of psychological risk factor. Her risk factors included being unhappy with pregnancy, being self-critical, and feeling stressed about being pregnant. Being self-critical during pregnancy is an important psychological risk factor. However, a 1999 study in the *Journal of Social and Clinical Psychology* indicated that while being highly self-critical might predict postpartum depression, you could moderate this factor by becoming strongly attached to your baby during your pregnancy.[12] Because of the resentment she felt toward herself and her baby, Carrie did not become attached to her baby while she was pregnant.

A research project at the University of Rochester School of Medicine studied 465 pregnant women from Wisconsin. Following these women at both one and four months postpartum, the study confirmed previous findings: That is, women who were depressed during pregnancy were also vulnerable to depression in the postpartum period. In addition, it was discovered that women who had thoughts of death and dying at the 30-day postpartum mark were still depressed by four months postpartum.[13] Although the risk of postpartum depression is first and foremost physical in nature, depression is a disorder that almost always has psychological as well as physical components to it.

One of the psychological factors that predispose you to postpartum depression is stress. As you know, perhaps only too well, becoming a new mother is stressful. And, perhaps not surprisingly, the thoughts and feelings you have about becoming a mother can also play a role in increasing your risk for postpartum depression. For instance, if you are excessively concerned about the healthy development of your baby, then you may be at risk for depression. A study done at Case Western Reserve University found that women preoccupied with the state of their baby's health were vulnerable to depression after giving birth.[14]

If you plan to return to work in the first few weeks or months after childbirth, there may well be stress related to childcare.[15] This kind of stress may not show up in the first few days or even weeks following the birth of your baby. It could take months before such stress begins to have an impact on your emotional health.

There is another kind of psychological distress that's related to becoming a new mother. This has to do with the role of parenting. Although it is easy to have fantasies about being a mother while you're still pregnant, the reality hits home when the baby arrives. That's when you discover that it's not glamorous to be on call 24 hours a day to a child that sleeps in short shifts, demands to be fed, and may cry constantly. Like many women, you may then begin to feel that you are inadequately prepared for parenting. Once you start to have feelings of incompetence as a new parent, depression may follow.[16]

Mothers today also have a great deal of conflict in deciding whether to be "stay at home moms" or return to their careers. Sometimes, you have no choice, as you may feel pressured by financial considerations. Other times, it may be related to your ambitions and dreams. Either way, deciding what to do and feeling caught in a bind can be added pressure that makes you more vulnerable to depression.

Other realities play a role in whether you become depressed. For instance, the temperament of your baby may not be what you expected. A whiney, overly active, and highly sensitive baby was probably not part of your plans for motherhood. So, if your baby's temperament is too far out of line from your expectations, then you can be at risk to become depressed.[17] In addition, a study reported in *Child Development* found that the degree of infant temperament difficulties was strongly related to a mother's level of postpartum depression.[18]

Clinicians and researchers usually say that negative or adverse life events can play an important part in the development of postpartum depression. Adverse life events are simply experiences that are traumatic or prolonged, such as divorce or the death of someone close. As such, they can cause prolonged psychological distress, which can trigger depression during or after pregnancy.[19]

Many women also experience considerable pain and anxiety during labor and childbirth. For some, the stress becomes so severe that a condition known as posttraumatic stress disorder (PTSD) can occur.

Renee, for example, had a relatively easy pregnancy. Labor was proceeding as she expected until her water broke. "The pain suddenly became so intense that everything I learned in Lamaze class meant nothing any longer," Renee remembers.

The doctor gave Renee medication through an IV, but this caused her heart rate to accelerate to a dangerous level. "All at once I was aware that there were doctors and nurses standing around me with panicked looks on their faces. I truly thought I was going to die," she says.

Vickie had a similar experience. She was scheduled for a caesarian section to deliver her son, Andy. "Soon after Andy was born, I started to feel sick," Vickie recalls. "I was shivering and the doctors and nurses were piling blankets on me. I guess my blood pressure started to drop because I remember a doctor saying there must be something wrong with the monitoring machine. When a nurse told him the machine was working fine, he called in other doctors. One of the doctors was squeezing an IV bag to get more medication in me. I kept thinking, 'I'm going to die.'"

Such extreme stress, resulting from a traumatic pregnancy, prolonged and intense labor, or a difficult delivery,[20] becomes part of your risk profile. Having posttraumatic stress disorder can be a trigger for the development of postpartum depression. A previous stressful event, such as physical, emotional, or sexual abuse at any previous time in your life, can also have a profound effect on the feelings you have about your own child[21] and may be associated with both depression and anxiety later in life.[22]

Other psychological risk factors you should be aware of include an unintended pregnancy, such as Carrie's, along with problems in the relationship between a woman and her own mother, ambivalence about pregnancy or conflict about becoming a mother, shortened hospital stays (which are common today), and physical problems experienced by your infant.

We recently asked a nurse practitioner who works in the neonatal intensive care unit at a large hospital how many of the mothers whose babies were in the intensive care unit soon after birth had, in her opinion, postpartum depression. She answered us with an astounding, "One hundred percent!" If you have a sick or physically challenged baby, it will likely be so traumatic for you that it will surely have a profound effect on your ability to cope with everyday life.

The happiness or unhappiness of your marriage can represent another important psychological risk factor for postpartum depression.[23] If you are unhappy with your marriage or your relationship with your partner, whether that involves communication difficulties, a lack of affection, dissimilarities of values, incompatibility in desired activities, or disagreements when it comes to making decisions, you become prone to experiencing postpartum depression.[24]

Prior to her pregnancy, Lucinda and her husband Jonathan argued regularly about finances and household chores. Jonathan accused Lucinda of spending too much money on clothes, and Lucinda complained that Jonathan left all the household chores for her to do. Things didn't improve when Lucinda got pregnant. "I cried because I was so happy when I found out I was pregnant," Lucinda says. "But Jonathan didn't react like I hoped he would. He seemed to be worried that this was going to be a drain on our financial resources." It was not surprising to us that Lucinda experienced postpartum depression.

A review of hundreds of research articles published in the *Canadian Medical Association Journal* in 1996 found that postpartum depression was most strongly associated with poor marital adjustment, recent life stressors, and depression during pregnancy.[25] If your marriage is rocky before your baby is born, you are likely to be depressed after delivery.

However, there's one other psychological factor that you should know about that is often overlooked—especially by mothers giving birth to a second child. That is, with your second child it will be the very first time you've given birth and gone home to raise both a newborn and another child. It's relatively easy for you to feel lost in the midst of what may sometimes feel like chaos. If you have difficulty coping with the strains of raising two or more children, this may throw you into a postpartum depression.

The Social Risk Factors

1. Lack of social and emotional support
2. Low socioeconomic status or unemployment

3. Being single or divorced
4. Low educational level
5. Pressure to breast-feed your baby

Besides the biological and psychological risk factors for developing postpartum depression, you have social risks as well. The most important social risk factor is a lack of social or emotional support, especially from your spouse or partner.[26] Because the transition to motherhood can be such a traumatic and demanding time, you need the help of others before, during, and after delivering your baby. In other words, you can't do it alone.

If you feel like you're doing it alone, then that in itself is related to an increased risk for postpartum depression.[27] In fact, past research shows that women have lower rates of postpartum depression when they say that they are cared for by partners, relatives, husbands, and friends.[28] In general, the wider the circle of people who are willing and able to help you, the less likely you are to suffer postpartum depression.[29]

When the father of your baby is not around enough, offers little emotional support, or fails to provide practical support, your chances of becoming depressed are increased. You will experience this feeling of being deprived of social support when you believe you are not receiving the amount of practical (baby-sitting, caregiving, or assistance with household chores) or emotional support you expected. A Danish study, reported in the *British Journal of Obstetrics and Gynaecology* in 2000, found that one out of three women who perceive themselves as social isolates will develop postpartum depression.[30]

Support is important not only during the postpartum period, but also during the birthing experience. For example, some evidence suggests that midwives and doulas can provide important, preventive support during delivery.[31] A doula is a woman who provides help and support during pregnancy and childbirth. Studies have shown that the constant support of a doula during labor improves the subsequent mental health of both mothers and their infants.[32] Similarly, if you have emotional support and comfort from your husband or partner, this will color how you feel about your delivery. Even your husband or partner's presence during childbirth positively influences whether you remember giving birth to your baby as pleasant or unpleasant.[33]

Many times we've found that new moms experience strong social pressure to nurse their babies. You may experience this kind of pressure from your doctor, nurses, family, friends, or even magazine articles. If you have any difficulty breast-feeding, if you don't want to breast-feed, or if you aren't physically able to breast-feed, you are likely to feel guilty and depressed. This, too, can be a factor in whether you feel depressed after giving birth to your baby. What often makes matters worse for you is that you may discover that your medical insurance policy will not cover the cost of a lactation consultant.

The reality of your life is intensely personal. That's why a variety of social circumstances can affect you during pregnancy or in the postpartum period. Such circumstances as having a low income, living in substandard housing, being unemployed, or even being a single or divorced mother can affect how you feel, the amount of social and emotional support you receive, and whether you will get depressed. Michael O'Hara, associate dean and professor at the University of Iowa's Department of Psychology and a researcher in postpartum depression, has concluded that socioeconomic factors, which include low education level and unemployment, contribute to depression "before, during and after pregnancy."[34]

Over the past twenty years, research has shown that social support promotes mental and physical well-being, especially during times of stress. The events following the tragic terrorist attacks of September 11, 2001, provide a good example of social support. People who experienced the loss of a loved one found that their social support network extended beyond family and friends to celebrities and strangers from all over the world who were there to provide physical, financial, and emotional support. On a smaller scale, we have seen the importance of so-cial support in women with risk factors for postpartum depression.

After Jane gave birth to her first child, her entire extended family took turns staying with her. They cared for Jane and the baby around the clock for several weeks, alternating shifts in order to assist her at a time of crisis because of her vulnerability to postpartum depression.

When Rebecca delivered her son, she and her husband were living in Alaska, where they had been transferred by the military three years pre-viously. For the two weeks following the birth of their son, the officers' wives club organized support in the form of nightly meal deliveries. Some of the wives even made special care packages with bath products. This embarrassed Rebecca's husband, who felt that outside help was unnecessary. But the support from the wives club was desperately needed by Rebecca, whose sense of isolation had been heightened by the absence of her own family, who lived a long way from Alaska. Her husband, who would not take time away from his duties in the military, had decided that neither of them should ask Rebecca's mother to visit, since traveling that far would be an emotional hardship. At a time when Rebecca needed a support system, she could only count on relative strangers.

We've frankly seen too many women with one of the many symptoms of a mood disorder during or following pregnancy who lacked social support, even within their own families. For instance, Katie, the mother of a new baby boy, recalled feeling all alone beginning in the hospital and lasting over the next few weeks following Stevie's birth. "I didn't feel that my husband was supportive," she says. "I came home from the hospital after the biggest event in my life, and he went back to work. He didn't act like my giving birth was a big deal. He was just anxious to get back to the office. I spent many days sobbing or talking on the phone to my sister in Cleveland."

All too often, women with risk factors for postpartum depression lack the necessary support from a partner or family and do not have trusting relationships with a church, work colleagues, or even their own physicians.

In summary, these risk factors—the biological, the psychological, and the social—tell you how likely you are to experience postpartum depression. Together with a measurement of the stress in your life, you can know if you are at risk for postpartum depression. Stress, itself, is a major risk factor. It is so important that we've devoted a later chapter (see Chapter 5) to a discussion of how stress and postpartum depression interact.

PART TWO

Make Sure You Get a Comprehensive Assessment for Postpartum Depression

4

What Is a Comprehensive Assessment?

POINTS TO PONDER IN THIS CHAPTER

- Unfortunately, there's no blood test or CAT scan for post-partum depression.
- A comprehensive assessment takes time and effort.
- There are questions you should ask and questions that should be asked of you during a comprehensive assessment.
- Good treatment may be compromised unless you first receive a comprehensive assessment.

If you are reading this chapter, it's likely that you have decided that you are at risk for postpartum depression or you are concerned that you already have it. Now you need to learn more about getting a comprehensive assessment. That, in fact, is the second key ingredient in the postpartum depression recovery program. This chapter will explain what a comprehensive assessment is, where you can get one, and what will happen in a comprehensive assessment.

What Is a Comprehensive Assessment for Postpartum Depression?

Until the day when we can rely on a simple blood test or a CAT scan or an MRI to diagnose postpartum depression, the best means for determining if you have postpartum depression is an assessment that is conducted on at least three levels. A comprehensive assessment will take into consideration your physical symptoms, your mood, and the social problems and stressors you may be facing. While it is certainly not a cut-and-dried test, an assessment isn't painful or invasive. But it will, however, require you to talk about yourself—physically and emotionally.

A comprehensive assessment is time-consuming. And if the assessment you're getting doesn't involve the ingredients we discuss in this chapter, you should be concerned about its thoroughness. The ideal postpartum depression assessment will involve the following steps:

1. Ruling out other possible medical conditions
2. A questionnaire
3. An interview and complete history

The comprehensive assessment will typically involve at least three professionals: a psychiatrist, a psychologist (or a social worker, nurse, or mental health counselor), and your obstetrician or primary care physician. Everyone on the team will assess a different part of your functioning. A team of postpartum depression specialists is in a much better position to address each of the three broad areas of concern in a thorough manner than just one professional or a physician who may not be trained as a specialist in postpartum depression.

You may question why you need a comprehensive assessment. You may say, "I already know I'm depressed, why do I need to go through all of this to have someone else tell me what I already know?" That's a fair question. The answer is that you may be depressed, but there may be more to the picture when you are pregnant or in the postpartum period. Consider what happened to Alexis:

After Alexis had her baby, she felt blue. That was followed by a foreboding sense of dread and anxiety. She had read about postpartum depression, and she was sure that's what she had. She scheduled an appointment with her physician. After listening to Alexis for a few minutes, he agreed that she was depressed and wrote out a prescription for an antidepressant.

Although Alexis filled the prescription, she didn't take the medication because she was concerned that it might affect her breast milk and be harmful for her baby. Her mood and low energy level didn't improve. Finally, taking the advice of a friend, she went to another doctor. "He did some tests and asked me lots of questions," Alexis said. "He found out I had diabetes and that was what was causing me to feel so awful."

A comprehensive assessment may reveal other serious disorders that can mimic depression but require far different treatment. If you receive a quick diagnosis, you may be treated for the wrong disorder—or you may receive the wrong treatment altogether.

Unfortunately, hasty diagnoses are just one of the problems we see. They are common practice because many professionals are overworked and short of time. A checklist or a brief interview often substitutes for a comprehensive assessment.

Because of publicity surrounding a few extreme cases of postpartum psychosis, women are diagnosing themselves and each other based on TV news reports or on magazine articles. Postpartum depression is so often talked about these days that many people lose sight of the fact that it is a serious condition needing proper diagnosis and treatment.

Ruling Out Other Possible Medical Conditions

Your physician can rule out other medical conditions that could be causing your symptoms. For instance, you could be experiencing a medication reaction.

Some medications can make you feel depressed. That is, the side effects of some medicines include depression. For example, if you took Tegretol (carbamazepine; a medication taken for control of seizures or to relieve certain kinds of pain), oral contraceptives, or Reglan (metoclopramide; a medication used to relieve nausea) over the previous year, it is possible that the depressed feelings or lethargy you may experience could be due to the side effects of these medications.

We see at least one person every month who has been referred for depression whose symptoms turn out to be due to the side effects of Reglan. Many women are prescribed Reglan or another metoclopramide during pregnancy for nausea and vomiting. For some of these women, the result of taking this medication is depression. However, once they come off metoclopramide, their depression vanishes.

Because there are several medications that can cause depression (including several of the birth control pills), make sure the doctor examining you knows what medications you've been taking over the past year.

Your depression could also be due to anemia. Anemia affects approximately three and a half million Americans, making it the most common blood disorder in the United States. The main symptoms of anemia are fatigue, weakness, and irritability, so you can see why it might be confused with postpartum depression. Anemia occurs when the amount of red blood cells or hemoglobin (a protein in the blood that carries oxygen) gets too low, causing body tissues to be deprived of oxygen-rich blood. When the blood can't carry oxygen to your organs, not enough energy can be produced for you to function normally.

The most common and severe type of anemia is iron-deficiency anemia. Just as the name implies, this form of anemia is due to insufficient iron. In the United States, 20 percent of all women of childbearing age have iron-deficiency anemia, compared with only 2 percent of adult men. The principal cause of this disorder in premenopausal women is loss of blood during menstruation. In fact, women lose up to 40 milligrams of iron each month during their menstrual cycle. However, other causes of anemia include eating inadequate amounts of iron-rich foods, a deficiency of vitamin B-12, a deficiency of folic acid, and poor iron absorption by the body.

Pregnant women are at increased risk of developing anemia. This is because the iron stores in the body can get depleted with the higher blood volume and demands of the fetus and placenta. After a delivery, the loss of significant amounts of blood can also lead to anemia. While anemia may interfere with your ability to do everyday chores or cause you to be too exhausted to enjoy either work or play, it can be distinguished from postpartum depression with a simple blood test, a physical exam, and a thorough medical history. The treatment of anemia can be simple, as well.

Another disorder that can either mimic or be associated with postpartum depression is thyroid disorder. From 4 to 10 percent of women develop a thyroid condition after having a baby. However, diagnosing a thyroid problem can be difficult because the thyroid gland secretions fluctuate.

The purpose of your thyroid gland is to make, store, and release thyroid hormones into your blood. Thyroid hormones control your body's metabolism. If you have too little thyroid hormone in your blood, your body slows down; too much in your blood and your body speeds up. When you are pregnant, your immune system—designed to fight infections—gears down. That is, your immune system gears down by no longer sending out signals to attack and destroy foreign cells, including bacteria and viruses, which are known as antigens. By suppressing this function, your immune system allows your baby to grow without being attacked—as though it were a foreign object. After you give birth, your immune system automatically gears back up again in order to fight infections in your body.

Sometimes, the immune system becomes overactive and begins attacking the thyroid gland, as if it were an antigen. When this happens, it results in postpartum thyroiditis. When postpartum thyroid dysfunction occurs, it will often reverse itself and return to normal functioning on its own. If dysfunction continues, you are likely to experience a rapid heartbeat, nervousness, and sweating. This condition can be treated with a synthetic thyroid hormone called levothyroxine sodium.

Diabetes is another disorder that needs to be ruled out during a comprehensive assessment. Approximately 3 to 5 percent of all pregnant women in the United States are diagnosed with *gestational diabetes,* a condition different from other forms of diabetes.

With other forms of diabetes, the pancreas fails to produce enough insulin, a hormone needed to convert sugar, starch, and other food into the energy needed to sustain life. Some of the common symptoms of diabetes are weight gain, increased fatigue, and irritability. If you have gestational diabetes, however, you have plenty of insulin. In fact, you may have more insulin in your blood than women who are not pregnant. However, the normal effect of insulin is partially blocked by a variety of other hormones, including estrogen, made in the placenta.

Most of the time, your pancreas will be able to make additional insulin to overcome this blocking effect. When your pancreas makes all the insulin it can, and there still isn't enough to overcome the effect of the placenta's hormones, gestational diabetes results. Generally, gestational diabetes disappears after you deliver your baby.

It is also possible that you may be suffering from an infectious disease, such as hepatitis, mononucleosis, or acquired immune deficiency syndrome (AIDS). All of these diseases have symptoms that include fatigue and low energy. Such symptoms can occur alongside depression, or they can be confused *with* depression.

Remember, just because you feel weak, sad, anxious, or fatigued, it doesn't necessarily mean that you have postpartum depression. You can't adequately diagnose yourself. However, because depression can be so painful and can cause you and your family so much suffering, even if you think you are sure you know why you are feeling depressed, fatigued, or anxious, be kind to yourself and obtain a comprehensive assessment.

A Questionnaire

A comprehensive assessment will involve a good screening tool or questionnaire, such as the Edinburgh Postnatal Depression Scale (EPDS). This questionnaire appeared in Chapter 2 for you to answer. If your score on the EPDS was between 10 and 12, we strongly advise you to proceed with a comprehensive assessment. If your score was 12 or more, a comprehensive assessment should be an immediate priority.

Keep in mind though that taking the EPDS is only a part of the assessment. It is not *the* assessment, although some physicians or mental health professionals may tell you it is. A screening device like the EPDS is just that—a screening tool. It simply indicates whether or not a more detailed evaluation should follow.

The Interview

Following your taking a depression screening instrument (and depending on your score), you should be interviewed by a member of the evaluation and assessment team. An interview is necessary to get to know you better. You will be asked about your physical and emotional symptoms, and when they started. You'll be asked about your family history and whether you have previously suffered from depression or any other psychiatric illnesses or mood disorders. You'll also be asked about your family life, including your marriage or current relationship, your family relationships, and your current level of stress and social support.

Furthermore, you can expect questions in the following areas:

- Your sleep patterns
- Your eating habits
- Your level of anxiety and depression
- Your thoughts (if any) about harming yourself or your baby
- Your experiences during pregnancy, labor, and delivery

If you get asked these and other questions, you can be more assured that you're in good hands. The interviewer, who may be a psychiatrist or another mental health professional, will ask you direct questions about your thoughts, behaviors, obsessions, and compulsions, and about previous psychiatric symptoms and treatment. Although these questions may be very probing and at times feel embarrassing, they are necessary to get a full picture of what you're going through.

Where Do You Go to Find a Postpartum Depression Team?

While the information in this book is designed to help you, only specialists in postpartum depression can make a definitive diagnosis and help you recover. Although any attentive doctor could determine that you are depressed by asking a few questions, only a skilled specialist will be able to definitively diagnose you and make treatment recommendations. But how do you find a postpartum depression team to obtain your comprehensive assessment?

You can ask your obstetrician, your primary care physician, or your baby's pediatrician for a referral to a postpartum depression specialist. You may also ask friends, especially a friend who has experienced postpartum depression. Furthermore, the obstetrics/gynecology department of a large hospital near you will either have a postpartum depression specialist on their staff or know of one. Finally, there are on-line resources, such as DepressionAfterDelivery.com, that maintain a list of specialists around the country. Seek out the help that you and your family deserve.

How Will You Know If the Professional You're Referred to Is a Postpartum Depression Expert?

Before you schedule an appointment with a specialist, here are some questions to ask:

- Do you specialize in treating postpartum depression, and if so, for how long?
- What percentage of your practice is related to women and mood disorders?
- Who are the other members of your assessment and treatment team?
- How do you conduct an assessment for postpartum depression?
- What is involved in the assessment? Will there be questionnaires and an interview?

Things to Keep in Mind About Your Assessment

The detection of postpartum depression is often complicated by several factors. For instance, if you're a first-time mother, you may not recognize that what you're feeling *isn't* normal. Also, because you will want to be a "good" mother, you may know something is wrong, but you may be hesitant to admit it out of a sense of shame, guilt, or fear of failing.

Furthermore, you may not know to whom you should turn if you're feeling anxious or depressed. It could be weeks before you are scheduled to see your obstetrician; you may not have a primary care physician; and you may feel like the pediatrician is focused on your baby. You could also be well beyond your postpartum six-week check and be feeling that you should be long past any postpartum problems.

Other factors that may complicate the diagnosis of postpartum depression have less to do with you and more to do with your physician. Often these days, doctors work very hard to care for many patients in a limited amount of time. That can mean that they may not have the time (or take the time) to ask you important questions that will give you a chance to express how you are feeling and coping. There are also many doctors who simply don't ask about a woman's quality of life.

There are also physicians who only feel comfortable with the "physi-cal" side of your condition. In other words, for some doctors, how you feel is less important than where you hurt.

Finally, a comprehensive assessment should result in a diagnosis and recommendations for treatment. It is very important that sufficient time be allowed for discussion of your diagnosis and proposed treatment. You should also feel more comfortable that a proper diagnosis has been made and that you are on your way to getting the right treatment.

5

What Is My Stress Level?

POINTS TO PONDER IN THIS CHAPTER

- Change always brings stress.
- Women are more likely to experience stressful life events than are men.
- Negative life events are risk factors for major depression.
- Stressful events predict postpartum depression.
- There is a strong connection between posttraumatic stress disorder and postpartum depression.

Whenever there is change in your life, you will also experience some stress. And literally any kind of change qualifies as a stressor—a change in your world to which you must adapt. In this chapter we will tell you how stress, as well as posttraumatic stress disorder, relates to postpartum depression. It is important in assessing your risk for postpartum depression to look carefully at how much stress there is in your life. It is also important to look back on traumas that you have experienced. During your comprehensive assessment, be sure that you share information about both recent and past traumas and stresses with the assessment team.

Grace had lived with George for three years when she became pregnant. She didn't want to have her baby without being married and

George agreed. "In a period of six weeks, we planned a full-blown wedding and reception for two hundred people," says Grace. "It was an extremely stressful time. After the wedding, we moved from a one-bedroom apartment to a house the same weekend I went into labor. I think I'm definitely a creature of habit and I'm sure all of these changes in such a short time contributed to my postpartum depression."

The stress of planning for a wedding, preparing for a baby, or moving to a new house can be exciting and thrilling. But stress can also cause problems. Stress can, for instance, lead to anxiety, an increase in your blood pressure, or depression. No matter how hard you work at avoiding it, one thing is certain: You can't avoid stress—and occasional trauma—in your life. The trick is to learn to cope with it without becoming depressed.

What Is Stress?

Although the concept of stress itself dates back to ancient Greece, we have come to think of it as a part of daily life. At least three-quarters of those who visit their doctors have a complaint related to stress.[1] Although you may use the word casually, stress is not to be underestimated. It plays a more powerful role than many people imagine. And it takes on a particularly powerful role during times of hormonal fluctuation, including pregnancy and the postpartum period. You are at increased risk for postpartum depression if you experience stress on a regular basis or have periods of acute stress.

Statistics tell us that if you suffer from depression, the chances are four out of five that your depression was brought on by some kind of stressful event in your life.[2] This is *especially* true if you are a woman. Women are actually three times more likely than men to experience depression in response to stressful events.[3]

Evolutionary biology has taught us that, centuries ago, our ancestors were constantly confronted by predators. They had to either fight or flee to survive. They also had to fight when hunting for food. So the stress response was as critical a bodily function as breathing. We believe this is why our bodies were designed to react to stress when physically threatened. In other words, our stress response system was originally designed for physical danger. However, the stressors we face today are very different and are primarily social and psychological. Nonetheless, the stress response is still adaptive in life-threatening situations. Unfortunately, because there are so many stressors you likely face day to day, your bodily defenses are probably often in a state of arousal. This will wear your body down over time.

Stress is a process that begins in your brain. What happens on a physical level is that when your brain senses change coming, an alarm goes off warning you of potential threat, and chemical messengers in the form of stress hormones are sent out to the various systems and organs of the body. This sets off a tidal wave of physiological changes. Heart rate, blood pressure, and muscle tension rise sharply. The stomach and intestines become less active, and the blood level of glucose (blood sugar) rises for quick energy. Your brain, in effect, arms your body for battle or escape. The stress hormones also activate cells in the immune system that rush to the battlefield to protect your body from whatever is threatening its stability. When the stressful event is over, your body returns to normal functioning. This, in essence, is what happens every time you experience change.

Your stress response is always active to some degree, which helps you deal with everyday changes in your environment. When you are presented with unusual, new, or excessive demands, challenges, or threats, the stress response readies your body for coping. But when life events or changes keep happening, or when multiple smaller stressors add up, you will experience chronic stress. And with each difficult life event, the brain struggles further to process what is going on. Eventually, your body begins to show the results of chronic stress as you develop anxiety, high blood pressure, sleep problems, or loss of appetite. When stress persists, the pathways of the brain become permanently altered. Almost any kind of stressful or difficult event or change will trigger the stress response—and that includes positive stress, like pregnancy and childbirth.

Positive stress is called *eustress* ("eu-" meaning "good," as in euphemism). It usually brings a wanted challenge, and its purpose is to keep us alert and interested in a task. This ultimately keeps us alive! We can feel eustress while mountain climbing, running a 5K race, or pursuing a favorite hobby. The key is that if your coping skills are greater than the challenge, you will feel positive stress. When the challenge is greater than your coping skills, you will feel *distress.*

It's very possible that you may live with so much stress in your life that you have stopped paying attention to both your brain's and body's signals warning you that you are not coping well. Here are some common signs that tell you there's too much stress in your life:

Physical Signs
- Heart palpitations
- Breathlessness, fast shallow breathing
- Dry mouth, "butterflies" in stomach, indigestion, nausea
- Diarrhea, constipation, flatulence
- Muscle tenseness, grinding of teeth
- Clenched fists, general muscle aches and pains
- Restlessness, hyperactivity, nail biting, finger drumming, foot tapping, hands shaking
- Fatigue, lethargy, exhaustion, sleep difficulties, headaches, frequent illnesses such as colds
- Sweaty or hot flushed feeling
- Cold hands and feet
- Frequent urination
- Overeating or loss of appetite

- Increased alcohol or tobacco use
- Loss of interest in sex

Mental or Psychological Signs

- Distressed, worried, upset, tearful, feelings of helplessness or hopelessness, hysterical, withdrawn, inability to cope, anxiety and depression
- Impatient, easily irritated and angry, frequent outbursts
- Frustrated, bored, guilty, insecure, fragile, low self-esteem
- Loss of interest in self-appearance and loss of interest in others
- Doing too many things at once, feeling rushed
- Failing to finish tasks
- Difficulty in thinking clearly, paying attention, concentrating, and making decisions; being forgetful and procrastinating
- Being accident-prone
- Feeling overwhelmed

These signs tell you that there is too much negative stress in your life or that your coping skills are not adequate to meet the challenges you face. Stress remains a risk factor for major depression and negative life experiences will precede depression about 80 percent of the time.[4]

Pregnancy and Stress

Cassie thought she couldn't get pregnant. "I was told by a doctor when I was a teenager that I could never get pregnant," Cassie says. "So my husband and I never used birth control. I never wanted children anyway, so it wasn't a problem for us. Until I got pregnant. Then, I couldn't stop crying. I didn't want a baby and I resented having to change my life."

Unlike Cassie, many women want to get pregnant and have a baby. However, even if you eagerly look forward to being pregnant, pregnancy brings with it major life changes. And changes—even positive, joyful ones—are stressful. Instead of pregnancy being that fabled time of emotional well-being, it is a critical life period with specific and unique stressors. However, this period of adjustment can be complicated when severe or unanticipated stress occurs.

Rhonda's story is a typical one we hear. "We had started renovating our house before I got pregnant and we had to continue in order to finish the house for the baby," Rhonda says. "Then, when I was three and a half months pregnant, I started getting sick every day and I was worried that there was something wrong with my baby. To top everything, my doctor ordered me to have complete bed rest for the last two months of my pregnancy. Talk about stress! I was really stressed out."

Serious or unexpected stress can include worrying about the physical changes you're going through, new and unanticipated medical problems, changes in your lifestyle, and worries about your job or career.

Carol had miscarried her first pregnancy after only eleven weeks. "When I got pregnant again six months later," Carol says, "I felt horrible for the first three months. Every day I had nausea, vomiting, headaches, and hot flashes. I was really scared I would miscarry again, but I didn't—I just felt anxious. The anxiety just kept getting worse throughout my pregnancy."

There are many things that can go through your mind during pregnancy. What's happening inside my body? Will I lose this baby? What if I miscarry? Is exercise healthy? What medications can I take? Did I do something before I knew I was pregnant that could cause harm to my baby?

And other stressors come into play, such as finances. If you're dependent on two incomes, you may get worried about the effects on your family if you have to stop working while you are pregnant. Your house can be a big stressor, too. You may want to decorate a room for the baby or even move to a bigger home. Things that would not have seemed so stressful before pregnancy take on more meaning when you are expecting a baby.

Your body image may also become an issue. Your clothes won't fit the same, but you may feel pressure to look professional at work. You may feel fat, and you may avoid sex. As your body expands, you may feel off balance much of the time. Movements that once came easily and naturally may have to be planned around a different center of gravity. Your body may feel alien and not quite yours any more.

If you've never been pregnant before, you may feel wonder at all the changes you're experiencing. And if you have been pregnant before, you may feel exhausted most of the time because you have at least another child to care for while you try to cope with all the other roles in your life. In short, pregnancy is likely to be a very stressful time in your life.

Childbirth

If you're like most women, by the ninth month of pregnancy you just want to begin labor and deliver your baby. While you may not look forward to childbirth, you know it's necessary in order to begin to love and care for your baby. However, there are aspects of labor and childbirth that can increase your risk for postpartum depression.

For instance, postpartum depression has been linked to the place and type of delivery you have, how much control you feel you have over the birthing experience, and your overall sense of satisfaction with the care and assistance you experience during delivery.

The type of delivery you have, whether caesarian or vaginal, may be related to depression afterward. You are more likely to be depressed if you give birth by a C-section as opposed to a vaginal delivery.[5] Furthermore, if you have a C-section delivery, having general anesthesia rather than an epidural will increase your risk for postpartum depression. Several studies have suggested that any obstetrical complications during labor or delivery may increase your risk for subsequent depression.[6]

Many women these days go to the hospital to have their babies with a "birth plan." In theory, this is a wonderful idea. We all know that if you rehearse something or know what to expect, you are likely to experience less stress. Hold on, though. There is a catch to this. When you have definite expectations—like those in a birth plan or wish list—then when things *don't* go the way you expect, it may be worse than it would have been if you'd had no expectations at all. One woman we know was so upset at how almost nothing went according to her birth plan that she always referred to it later as that "stupid birth plan."

If you like your obstetrician and feel supported by the nurses and doctors during your delivery and hospital stay, and if they make you an active part of the delivery experience, you are less likely to develop postpartum depression. If you do get it, you may have a milder case than another woman who disliked her obstetrician, was neglected by staff, and not informed about what was happening. The amount of information you are given prior to going to the hospital, and the communication you experience during labor and delivery with the hospital staff, will help you feel that you have some control. Having a measure of control over your labor and delivery will reduce your risk for postpartum depression.

Another aspect of stress during childbirth is that of pain and the expectation of pain. A part of the brain called the hippocampus mediates between the expectation of an experience and the reality of that experience. When major differences arise, your central nervous system is activated. When this happens, it could lead to birth complications, including having your contractions stop.[7]

Childcare After Delivery

Once you've given birth, then there are other stressors that can affect you. Most of these new stressors, as you might expect, have to do with the care of your baby. For example, breast-feeding can be a major stressor for you. As we discuss in Chapter 8, your decision to breast-feed and even whether you can breast-feed or not can be very stressful to you and how you view yourself as a woman and as a mother.

And then there are childcare concerns. Worries and problems related to the care of your baby have consistently been found to be risk factors for the development of postpartum depression. The stress of a long and difficult labor and the stress of a traumatic delivery can sometimes seem less daunting than the many challenges, and the accompanying stress, of being a new mother.

What if your baby has a difficult temperament? That's a stressor that can increase your chances of developing postpartum depression.[8] When children are irritable, fussy, overly active, or chronically distressed, your feelings of competence as a mother will slowly erode. Furthermore, a temperamental baby will cause you to respond differently than you might to a placid, calm infant. When your self-esteem as a parent begins to slip away, you may not try as hard, you may feel tired more often, or you may respond with fewer smiles and be less playful with your baby.[9] In other words, you will develop more ambivalent feelings toward your baby. This is especially likely to happen if you are an adolescent mother or if your baby was the result of an unplanned pregnancy.[10]

Learning to care for a new baby, adjusting to the infant's sleep schedule, and settling into all the new routines a baby requires, in addition to childcare arrangements, all require extraordinary coping skills. It's even more complicated if you gave birth to twins or triplets.

Denise found this out when she had triplets and developed postpartum depression as well. "It's overwhelming knowing that when you do what you don't feel like doing," Denise says, "that you have to do it times three. I also realized how difficult it was to do some of the things that were so easy before—like go to the store for a gallon of milk. Now, it involves dressing three children, putting them in three car seats, and hauling a big stroller around. It's a monumental task to do everyday errands."

Another major stressor is being pregnant when you already have children at home—especially one or more toddlers. You may feel fatigued, but you won't be able to get the rest you did when you had just a baby. You may fear how you will handle two or more children. You may fear failure, and you may fear that you've made a mistake by getting pregnant. Every worry is a stressor. And every added stressor will make you more vulnerable to postpartum depression.

Posttraumatic Stress Disorder

Christina had a very difficult delivery. "I started feeling contractions one morning about a week before my baby was due," Christina says. "I laid on the couch for several hours and then went to my scheduled doctor's appointment that afternoon. By that time, the contractions were coming every four to five minutes and I was doubled over with pain."

When she got to her appointment, the doctor told her she was only dilated to one centimeter. "He sent me to the hospital," Christina recalls, "and I was hooked up to a fetal monitor and contraction monitor and for the next several hours they watched me. But I was in intense pain. I begged for an epidural, but they told me that any pain medication would slow down the contractions and stall my progress."

The pain, Christina remembers, was "indescribable." She says she suffered this pain for almost 24 hours before she was given medication. "It was," she now says, "worse than anything I could ever have imagined."

When Christina came home from the hospital with her baby, she was depressed and anxious. She was often unable to sleep—even when her baby rested. When she did fall sleep, she frequently awoke with a start, feeling like she was back in the delivery room, dying.

Posttraumatic stress disorder (PTSD), first defined in 1980 to describe long-standing symptoms that follow trauma, can be the result of being exposed to an event that causes real or threatened death or serious injury, or it can come from witnessing an event that involves death, injury, or harm to another person. The concept came from the experiences of Vietnam veterans. Later, it was expanded to include abuse, rape, torture, being the victim of a crime, being in or witnessing a horrific accident, or being trapped in a fire. You can also experience PTSD by having a traumatic labor or delivery.

Just because you experience a traumatic event, it doesn't mean you will develop PTSD. The likelihood of getting PTSD depends on whether or not you have been through trauma before, whether you have had a mood disorder in the past, and what happens during your pregnancy, labor, and delivery. If you have preexisting emotional or psychological problems, you are naturally more susceptible to having any new trauma result in a recurrence of the old traumatic event.

So, just as chronic stress can play a major role in your having postpartum depression, traumatic experiences can do the same.[11] Research consistently shows that difficult life events—traumatic episodes—trigger depression just as often as chronic stress. And this is true at any time from well before you get pregnant, during pregnancy, during delivery, or in the first year of raising your new baby.[12]

What is a trauma for you can vary. Traumatic events can range from discovering you are pregnant to being ill during pregnancy; from domestic violence and marital problems to the loss of a job or the death of someone close to you; from a traumatic delivery to a medical emergency for your baby. If you have experienced a trauma, and if you have ever suffered from PTSD, you need to tell someone during your assessment.

Coping with Stress

You may feel at this point that you have little or no control over the stress you feel. Nothing could be further from the truth. If you have been under a great deal of stress, suffer from chronic stress, or have been through past or recent trauma, we strongly encourage you to tell your assessment team about this. However, there are ways to prepare yourself to deal with future stressors, or in the words of some psychologists, to "inoculate" yourself against stress.

Here are a number of strategies that can help you reduce the effects of stress or increase your ability to cope.

- Listen to your body. Pay attention to your intuition.
- Remember that nine things out of every ten we worry about are things that will never happen. Save your coping energy for the tenth.
- Fake it till you make it. You may not feel strong enough to cope successfully, but until you are ready, just fake it—especially with your baby.
- Check yourself when feeling stressed. Watch your individual stress level.
- Balance rest and activity.
- Learn how to relax. Learn relaxation strategies for use during the most stressful times.
- Exercise regularly. Exercise burns up excess adrenaline and normalizes endorphins, the body's natural morphine-like chemicals.
- Avoid sugar and eat a balanced diet.
- Learn about the mental tool of "thought stopping" or find something physically or mentally to replace worried thoughts.
- Decrease the demands on your body.
- Avoid negative and critical people.

There is also evidence that social support and healthy coping responses have a positive effect on stress during pregnancy. Chapter 11 will tell you how to increase your social support network.

Your Assessment and Stress

Finally, stress is a significant factor in determining whether you will become depressed, and if so, how severe your level of depression will be.

Make sure you find support and mobilize a support system. Make sure that your assessment and treatment team know the extent of stress in your life. Don't let your pride or the fact that you have always been a strong, successful woman stand in the way now. Treatment is just a step away. However, it often takes incredible strength to do what needs to be done. Being treated for postpartum depression is no exception. We know you can meet this challenge.

6

Roadblocks to Successful Treatment

POINTS TO PONDER IN THIS CHAPTER

- There may be several things that block you from getting the treatment you need.
- One important roadblock to treatment is denial.
- Fear is a hindrance to treatment for many women with postpartum depression.
- Overcoming these common roadblocks is a key to beginning treatment.

Now that you've had a complete assessment, you've also received a diagnosis along with treatment recommendations. Two possibilities exist: One, you were told that you don't have postpartum depression; or two, you were told you do have postpartum depression and need treatment.

If you received the news that you're experiencing postpartum depression, then you may be heaving a big sigh of relief—at least you have a diagnosis. On the other hand, if you were told that you have postpartum depression, you may be wondering what will happen next. You may also be worried about treatment. In fact, you may be reluctant to accept the treatment recommendations you were given. We've learned that some women with postpartum depression have certain roadblocks—some personally imposed and some thrust upon them by others—that interfere with their treatment. You will learn in this chapter about the various roadblocks that may make successful treatment difficult to start.

You may be very anxious to accept treatment and get on with getting help. However, we urge you not to skip over this chapter as some of the issues we will discuss may relate to you—if not now, perhaps in the future as you proceed with treatment.

Why You Might Avoid Treatment for Postpartum Depression

"I remember thinking, this isn't right," Mary told us. She looked awkward and embarrassed as she told us she had heard of postpartum depression, but "I didn't want it and I can't even imagine that I might have it—or that it might have me."

Mary added that she had been "faking it" with her husband, her friends, and her children. However, she said she couldn't fake it any longer. "I felt constantly overwhelmed and annoyed by my 3-year-old son. I was always putting him off and that wasn't fair to him. I realized when his behavior became worse that I was hurting my child by not feeling good enough to play with him or show him affection."

It took Mary five months into her second pregnancy before she called her obstetrician and told him she was having panic attacks at least twice a day. "I only asked for help when the behavior of my 3-year-old began to change," Mary told us. "About the same time, my husband started becoming distant and pleading with me to stop yelling all the time. It wasn't just about me any more."

One of the most important reasons for *not* putting off treatment is because your baby and your other children will suffer when you are depressed. But it's not just your children who will be affected by your depression. So will your family and friends.

The words we hear over the telephone the most are, "My family thinks I need help." Our response is usually, "What do *you* think?"

Often, we sense a woman's struggle with the answer. We believe that women struggle with this question because by acknowledging they need help means they are giving up a measure of control in their lives. The women we meet are typically strong women who have run their families, their jobs, large departments, and even corporations. They have been the ones to whom their friends and family have turned when help was needed. And they have always somehow been in control and on top of things at home, at work, and in the community. However, when they come to our office, they are often like Joanne.

Joanne, the project manager for a big computer company, was used to being in charge of groups of people and she was accustomed to success. She prided herself on her ability to work long hours and to get multi-million dollar projects done on time. When she came to see us shortly after the birth of her daughter, she wanted us to know she wasn't herself lately. "Some days I can barely figure out how to take a shower and plan a bath for my baby," she said. "I used to be the champion multi-tasker. Now I just feel overwhelmed with the simplest tasks."

Yolanda, who was 19 years old when she came to see us, shared her hesitation toward seeking treatment with our team. "It's hard being a young woman, trying to prove to everyone that you are an adult and in control of your own life, and then losing that control," she said. "By coming forward to get help, you have to admit to yourself and your family that you are not as strong as you thought you were."

She said she waited several months before she sought help. "No matter how bad things got, I told myself that I alone had to handle it," Yolanda said. "I kept thinking, 'What if I went to the doctor and he told me that I needed to be on medication. That means I'm crazy and I know I'm not crazy. I am just a little depressed.'"

Many women, by admitting they need help, are like Mary, who had wanted to tough it out and "Not give in to this awful postpartum thing." On the other hand, there is a stigma related to any kind of emotional or psychological problem. By going for treatment, you run the risk of being stigmatized and seen as being weak or "disabled."

Like many women we know, you might think it was better in the past when there was a shroud around depression and anxiety disorders associated with pregnancy and the postpartum period. That is, you may feel that somehow it was better before Andrea Yates.

That's because Andrea Yates sensationalized the word "postpartum." It was reported that Mrs. Yates, the Texas mother who drowned her five children in 2001, had, among many other serious problems, postpartum psychosis. One woman in a thousand gets postpartum psychosis. But nearly every woman who seeks help with postpartum depression now feels the stigma. When Sharon was diagnosed with postpartum depression, her husband asked her if that meant that he now had to be afraid for the safety of his child.

Yolanda, like Joanne and like Sharon, was more than a little depressed. All three women had lived with postpartum depression for weeks and months before admitting that they had a problem, and that they had to ask for help. "Maybe I could have done this alone," Mary said after she received treatment and her symptoms disappeared, "but I learned that you don't have to do it alone. I am no longer embarrassed to admit that there are people out there who can help me feel better and function better. It is amazing how you don't realize how bad you really feel until you feel better."

Another reason why you might try to avoid treatment for postpartum depression is because of your concerns about taking medication. "The first time I had postpartum depression, I would say it wasn't severe, but it was pretty bad, and I resisted taking medication," Patty said. "I was afraid it would make me feel spacey. You see things on television about people in mental hospitals, and you don't want to be like that. You're just having a baby."

Patty said she was frightened by commercials on television that announced that one of the possible side effects of taking Prozac could be a reduction in her sex drive ("Like I had any to begin with," she quipped). She also remembered news reports claiming that actor Phil Hartman was killed by his wife because she had been taking Zoloft. "What if it makes me want to kill? Is that supposed to make me want to take Zoloft?" Patty asked.

Jill came to see us after her second delivery and after getting seriously depressed for the second time. "Even though this was my second bout with postpartum depression, I still fought with my team about taking medication," Jill says, looking back on her treatment. "But they didn't give up on me. Everyone listened to me—and to my reluctance to being on medication."

What Are the Roadblocks to Treatment?

The most significant roadblocks to treatment are:

1. Denial
2. Guilt
3. Self-reliance
4. Fear
5. Noncompliance with treatment advice
6. Systemic problems

Why do we see these six items as roadblocks? Because they can prevent you from getting or accepting the kind of help you need at one of the most critical points in your own and your family's lives. If you have postpartum depression, you need treatment. You can't take the chance that you will become seriously depressed. Nor can you risk the health and well-being of your baby.

Denial

The first possible roadblock to you receiving treatment for your depression is denial. Despite having a comprehensive assessment and a diagnosis of postpartum depression, you may hold out the belief and hope that the experts made a mistake and you do not really have postpartum depression. In fact, you may insist to yourself that you don't have it and you don't want it.

"None of this was the way I planned," said Nicole, a 24-year-old mother of a 6-month-old boy. "It wasn't supposed to be like this. I didn't plan for it to be anything but wonderful and a loving, happy time in my life. I don't want to think I'm depressed because I gave birth to a beautiful son."

You may deny you are depressed or you may deny you need treatment. Like Nicole, you could say, "Women have been having babies for centuries, so it's no big deal. I *can't* be depressed!"

While depression wasn't in your plans, it's important to stop fighting the idea that you are depressed and accept the diagnosis and treatment. You will have to accept one important reality: by engaging in treatment you must give up the fantasy that your pregnancy and delivery were the happiest times of your life. For you—as for many others—this is just a fantasy.

Finally, the most serious problem with maintaining your denial is that it prohibits you from getting the treatment you need to make life livable for you, your baby, and your partner.

Guilt

Guilt and shame go together as twin roadblocks that can prevent you from entering into treatment. As much as we would like to think that we live in an enlightened twenty-first century, the fact is that psychological problems and treatment for "mental disorders" are still often regarded as stigmas.

Elaine learned this when she was pregnant and talking with her mother-in-law. "We were having a discussion about women who have postpartum depression after the Andrea Yates case was on the news,"

Elaine says. "She told me that she didn't believe in postpartum depression. My mother-in-law actually said postpartum depression is the latest 'in' disease and that it is fashionable for women to claim they have it. I knew if I ever felt depressed I could never tell her."

Dr. Kay Jamison, professor of psychiatry at the Johns Hopkins School of Medicine, wrote *An Unquiet Mind,* a book in which she described her depression. She said that talking openly about her depression brought out a "darker side of human nature" and that her disclosure almost cost her her position. "What haunted me the most, however, was the hundreds of letters and telephone calls from people who felt they could never be honest about their mental illness," Jamison said, "because if they did they would lose their jobs, friends, or health insurance. They wrote over and over again that it was hard to be honest about mental illness when their hospital privileges, medical licenses or academic degrees were at stake."[1]

Mary Lou, a woman with postpartum depression, told other women in group therapy the shame she felt about having depression. "Who can you tell?" she asked. "If I told my mother, she would look down on me as if I were weak and unappreciative of the beautiful baby that I have. But I'm tired of hiding in my house and not letting anyone know what I'm going through. I just don't want to feel guilty anymore."

Often, if you keep hiding your postpartum depression from others, the anxiety and fears of talking about your depression will just increase. Coming to grips with your shame and guilt and telling people usually eases the burden. It's often a relief to begin telling others and talking about what you're doing to get better.

Self-reliance

We've already mentioned in other chapters that many of the women we see with postpartum depression have been independent, self-reliant women. While there's something admirable about self-reliance and while being fiercely independent can be a strength in the business world or the arts, it can play havoc with you when you have postpartum depression and need to ask for help.

Dana had worked her way to an executive producer position with a talk show in a large-market television station. She was proud of the fact that she had done this all on her own and she had become successful because of her hard work and determination. However, when she decided she was secure enough to get pregnant and take a few weeks off to have a baby, she was confronted by postpartum depression. "I was determined that I could fight this demon on my own," she said. "I'd always fought my own battles, I was proud of never needing to talk to others about my problems, and there I was caught between my need to do it again on my own and my dawning recognition that this was a fight I couldn't win by myself."

Dana resolved this by following the advice given at the end of her assessment and tentatively going for a first therapy appointment. "You don't know how hard this is," she said to the therapist on the first visit. "I don't want to be here and I still think that if you just tell me what to do I can solve this problem by myself."

Self-reliance is not a bad trait in a country that treasures self-reliant people. However, treatment requires you to ask for help and then follow the suggestions of others. And you must acknowledge that these professionals know more than you about postpartum depression and its effective treatment.

Fear

Of all the potential roadblocks to treatment, perhaps the most essential one is fear. Consider the fears that may confront you as you weigh the various recommendations made at the end of your assessment.

You may fear—

- that if you talk about your real thoughts and fantasies your baby may be taken from you;
- that friends and family will not understand what you're going through;
- that medication will hurt you or your baby;
- that you may become dependent on any medication you're prescribed;
- that you may learn things about yourself that are frightening;
- that therapy will somehow damage your relationship with your husband or partner.

These are all fears that we've heard women talk about and share with us and with other women in group therapy.

"If I told you the thoughts I have about my baby," Marilyn said in her third therapy session, "I'm afraid you'd call protective services and have my baby taken away."

In Chapter 2 we described one category of postpartum depression in which there are obsessive thoughts. Although you are not likely to have a serious mental disorder, you may still have frightening and bizarre thoughts about yourself and your baby.

For example, Lorraine anxiously confessed that she had images of hurting her baby. "Of course, I'd never do anything to hurt her," Lorraine said. "I just have weird thoughts about my baby being hurt by me. Am I crazy?"

You are not crazy because you may have strange or terrifying thoughts that you can't seem to shake. Telling your postpartum depression team about these thoughts will not lead to your baby being taken from you nor to you being "locked up." In our experience, these are fairly "normal" and typical for you to have, particularly if you have a serious case of postpartum depression. We have never taken a baby away from a mother with postpartum depression; nor have we ever recommended this. We have also never seen a woman who harmed her baby after she told a skilled professional about these thoughts or obsessions.

Instead, what we have seen is that when you are able to talk about these thoughts, then we are able to most appropriately see that you get the kind of treatment that will reduce or eliminate such worrisome thoughts.

Another common fear is that your husband, your family, or your friends will not understand what you're going through. Unless they've experienced postpartum depression, the chances are that they won't truly understand how you have suffered. However, you can help to increase their understanding by talking about your feelings as well as your treatment. We often encourage women to bring family and friends to group therapy sessions so they get to hear from other women and their families what postpartum depression is and how treatment can be successful.

Another major but common fear is that you will be prescribed medication. Along with this are additional fears— that medication will hurt you or your baby and that you may become dependent on any medication you're prescribed. As with other fears, it is important that these be shared with the postpartum assessment and treatment team. When you share these with your team, then they can address these concerns with you and together plan how your fears can be relieved and taken into consideration through treatment. These fears will be addressed more in Chapters 7 and 8.

The other fears that are frequently expressed by women are that you may learn things about yourself that are frightening or that therapy may somehow damage your relationship with your husband or partner. If you've never been in psychotherapy or counseling before, you may have some misconceptions about what will happen there.

We will describe psychotherapy in more detail in Chapter 9; however, here it is important for you to bear in mind what the goals and directions of treatment will be. If you have been referred for psychotherapy because of postpartum depression, then certainly working with your therapist to find ways of reducing and eliminating your symptoms will be very important. Furthermore, you and your therapist will examine aspects of your life that may need revision or alterations in order for you to feel less depressed. Your therapist won't tell you what to do or what to change. However, together you will be able to explore and agree on steps that are likely to be in your best interest.

Noncompliance with Treatment Advice

An important roadblock to successful treatment is your reluctance or inability to follow the recommendations of your postpartum team. Reluctance to follow suggestions and prescriptions from a treatment team or doctor can come in many forms.

For instance, there is research showing that if you are depressed you are three times more likely to ignore your doctor's instructions, even when you have voluntarily gone for help.[2] "The problem of noncompliance is quite large," says Robin DiMatteo, professor of psychology at the University of California at Riverside. "Overall, about 40 percent of people leave their doctors' offices and do not follow recommendations." DiMatteo is talking about patients in general. If you're depressed, it may be even harder to follow a doctor's advice.

This is not because you are against following the advice of others. And this is not because you don't want to get better. The reason we think women with postpartum depression sometimes have difficulties following our recommendations is because often with pregnancy and the prospect of having a child your expectation for joy and happiness is so high. Having your expectations and dreams shattered can make you feel overwhelmed and even immobilized.

Leslie was told she needed medication as well as individual psychotherapy. "I'm not sick," she told her husband after she was told what the recommendations following the assessment were. "Isn't depression just a state of mind that can be changed at will?" she asked him. "Maybe if I'm just stronger and believe in myself more, I won't have to take medication or see the psychologist."

Unfortunately, her husband and family reinforced this belief. As a result, Leslie suffered needlessly for two additional months before she agreed she couldn't get better on her own.

Many people do go against the suggestions and advice of their doctors and their treatment team. If you've had a comprehensive assessment and you've been afforded the best possible advice, then you should accept that the experts know how you're going to get better as quickly as possible.

Systemic Problems

It's not *your* system that is likely to be a roadblock to treatment but rather the environmental and health care system. We can handle your system; however, the social and medical system is sometimes difficult to navigate.

There are many good, competent doctors in this country. There are great obstetricians, wonderful, caring family physicians, terrific internists, and sensitive pediatricians. However, there are also doctors who are overworked and far too busy who are frequently not able to take the time to listen to you or ask you how you're feeling. There are also physicians who know little about postpartum depression. Or worse, only know what they learned many years ago. We still hear about doctors who don't understand postpartum depression, think that all depression is the maternity blues, and advise all of their patients to wait a few weeks and see if they don't get better on their own.

You may also be in a medical group in which some physicians are sensitive, caring, and able diagnosticians, while others (who might be on call when you need help) will not be right for you when you are depressed.

Our advice is to change doctors or make sure you make an appointment with the right doctor for you—the one who will listen carefully and seriously to your symptoms and do what is best for you.

Another systemic problem relates to the health care insurance and disability insurance organizations. As medical and mental health professionals, we have to deal with the insurance companies and the offices that approve disability coverage. Needless to say, we have encountered wide variability in the eagerness and willingness to help women who need approval for treatment, hospitalization, or disability leaves. So often the most recalcitrant and stubbornly unhelpful people have been those who appear more interested in saving their company a few dollars than taking the needs of depressed women into consideration.

Although we recognize that many people who have the responsibility of approving inpatient and outpatient psychological and medical help are decent, hardworking professionals, there are some bad apples, too. There are those health care gatekeepers who aren't supportive of women with postpartum depression and can be hostile and petty when it comes to professional recommendations for the women who have *paid* for their insurance.

For instance, Ruth had a wonderful pregnancy up until her sixth month, when she was hit from the rear by another car and pushed completely under a truck. She was so traumatized physically and emotionally that she was put on psychiatric medications and told not to return to work because of her high levels of anxiety. One month later, she delivered her son—all three pounds of him—in an emergency caesarian section when his heart rate showed that he was in distress.

Ruth's son was in the Neonatal Intensive Care Unit for about three weeks. She lived in a daze during that time. When he came home, her employer of ten years began to call her, questioning her disability. She was asked many questions about the fact that her postpartum depression team had placed her on total disability. Ruth told us, "As soon as I said I couldn't get behind the wheel of a car because I freaked out, they took the ball and ran with it. They told me that not driving was not a covered benefit of my disability policy and that someone could drive me to work."

Her psychologist made several phone calls to Ruth's disability company. The woman who handled disability claims challenged her diagnoses of posttraumatic stress disorder and postpartum depression, and insisted that Ruth return to work immediately—against the advice of her entire postpartum depression team.

Ruth's story is all too common in our experience. We have worked with women who were illegally let go from their jobs because they requested a disability leave after a diagnosis of postpartum depression. And we've worked with mothers who were not allowed back into teaching jobs because an administrator in a school board office determined that a woman with postpartum depression "shouldn't be around children."

Because these kinds of problems exist, it is all the more reason to work with a skilled and experienced postpartum depression treatment team. Most of us have encountered every kind of problem or situation there is. We are in a much better position to fight the system than you are. Dealing with the system is the job of your treatment team.

In conclusion, we have presented various roadblocks to you getting into and benefiting from treatment from a postpartum treatment team. Having been prepared by becoming aware of these potential hindrances to treatment, you are ready to get the treatment you need. Part Three tells you more about why you need a treatment team and what to expect from each member of the team.

Receive Multi-dimensional Treatment from a Specialized Postpartum Depression Team

7

Why Do I Need Treatment from a Postpartum Depression Team?

POINTS TO PONDER IN THIS CHAPTER

- Do not delay treatment.
- Many women with postpartum depression avoid treatment for various reasons.
- Without treatment, your postpartum depression may not improve or may get worse.
- A specialized postpartum depression treatment team can address all areas of causes and risks for your depression.

The third key ingredient in our proven recovery plan is to get good treatment. In this part of the book you will learn more about the kinds of treatment that we have found are essential for you to conquer postpartum depression. We describe here in detail the specific types of treatment we use and recommend for our patients. Treatment approaches covered in this section of the book will include those that are medical, psychological, social, and parenting-related. Furthermore, we will review alternative forms of therapy that are often used or preferred by other doctors, therapists, and women who are suffering from postpartum depression.

Keep this important point in mind as you read the next several chapters: Our most important advice to you is to get help from a team of experts in postpartum depression. And the sooner you do that, the sooner you will recover. However, many women with postpartum depression avoid good treatment.

Why You Need Treatment

If you have postpartum depression, we believe there are several reasons why you need treatment. You, like a great many other women with postpartum depression, will not improve without treatment. In fact, you may get worse. If you get worse, this has significant consequences for you, your baby, and your family.

If you get more depressed, you could become suicidal. The threat of suicide is of major significance for you and your family. Even if you don't become suicidal, though, you will continue to be depressed. And this, too, has a serious impact on your family. Untreated and prolonged depression can lead to psychological, social, and academic consequences for your child (this will be discussed in more detail in Chapter 12). Furthermore, your depression can lead to marital problems and isolation from friends and family, as well as decreased efficiency in your job and the potential for loss of income due to disability later on.

But there are also other serious repercussions for you when your depression goes untreated. There can be increased stress on both your body and your brain. Researchers have found that prolonged, serious depression can lead to a type of permanent brain damage in several areas of the brain. This results in future episodes of depression being triggered by less serious and more frequent events in your life.

The bottom line is that without treatment, your life can become one of distance and dread. You will be distanced from your children and those who love you. And you are likely to dread the possibility of future depressive episodes. Even if you are a strong woman who does make it through the experience without help, you will have permanently altered pathways in your brain and be even more susceptible to stressors and hormonal events in the future. With the right treatment, however, there is tremendous hope of recovery and the avoidance of most or all of these potential consequences.

Why You Need a Postpartum Depression Treatment Team

Our team, as you know by now, consists of a psychiatrist and two psychologists. One psychologist specializes in helping women and their families with depression during and after pregnancy, and the other helps parents improve their parenting and discipline skills. We believe strongly in the team approach. The women we help also believe in the team approach. The reason is not complicated. The team approach works!

Why do you need a physician, especially one who is skilled in psychopharmacology, along with a psychotherapist and a parenting advisor besides your obstetrician or family practitioner?

This approach works for several reasons. (1) There are several risk factors and causes of postpartum depression and these risks have to do with your biology, your psychology, your social support network, and your parenting skills. It is unlikely that one person, particularly your obstetrician or family physician, can treat all of these areas. (2) Medication will likely be an important cornerstone in your treatment and only an expert in psychopharmacology and postpartum depression will be able to determine the most appropriate medication. (3) Your physician is unlikely to be able to provide the individual and group treatment that you need. (4) There are few experts in parenting and postpartum depression. In order to minimize the effect of depression on your baby and other children, you need the help of a specialist in parenting.

The Psychotherapist's Role

If you're getting treatment from a team, then for that team to function well, there must be a "quarterback." Having strong family support or a caring husband can't take the place of a quarterback because they don't know the playing field.

What role will a psychotherapist play? The psychotherapist will call the signals for treatment and make sure the treatment is coordinated. In addition, the therapist who coordinates the team approach will provide individual and/or group treatment for you. But the work of the therapist goes beyond even this. The therapist will certainly be an expert in the treatment of postpartum depression, but she will facilitate coordination between all team members, for instance, by maintaining 24-hour, round-the-clock communication with the psychiatrist.

By having more contact with you than anyone else on the team, the therapist will help you to feel comfortable talking about issues that are difficult to talk about. And seeing you often and for long periods of time means that the therapist can catch you at many different "moments in time," so she gets a more rounded and fuller picture of you.

Think of the psychiatrist as the team's "coach." In our experience, he or she plans the overall strategy. But he needs the best information to do that, and for this he relies on the therapist. His scope is that of the big picture—re-regulating your brain chemistry so symptoms decrease and daily functioning improves. The therapist deals with the details, and this requires more time and attention—and that's why practicing psychotherapy is different than reviewing your medication treatment.

That is not to say that a psychiatrist can't or shouldn't do psychotherapy. But women need to be proactive and ask whether they are getting psychotherapy from their psychiatrists. If they are in the psychiatrist's office for less than 45 minutes, it's not considered psychotherapy.

The therapist's role begins by coordinating the team. Just as football teams practice and have a game plan, good medical team coordination is essential. Team members will have frequent and constructive communication among themselves. This way, when you hide how you are feeling from one team member, chances are that you've told another one how you feel. This kind of coordination improves our success rate.

What Degree Should a Psychotherapist Have?

We don't believe that it will make a difference in your treatment whether a therapist has a master's degree or a doctorate, or if it's a degree in psychology, social work, counseling, or nursing. What is important is that this person has been trained out of the classroom by, and continues to work with, a medical doctor who specializes in postpartum depression.

More Than 9 to 5 Availability

On any given Saturday night, each member of our team is likely to get paged at least once. Often, that results in team members consulting with each other. Such availability can be a crucial lifeline to you; you shouldn't be told to wait until Monday or to go to the emergency room. Postpartum depression doesn't lend itself to that kind of "working hours" treatment.

Lucy paged her psychologist, sobbing. "I feel terrible," she said. "I stopped taking my medications three days ago. I'm only 24 years old, and I don't want to be taking pills."

Lucy's psychologist was concerned about her, and she also knew that medication issues need to be handled by the psychiatric team member. She asked Lucy if she would page the psychiatrist, and Lucy continued to cry. The psychologist phoned the psychiatrist to get medical advice, and communicated the information to Lucy, as well as helping Lucy realize that in order for the team to help her, she had to make decisions about medication with her medical doctor. Lucy certainly could have talked to any one of the team members about her feelings about taking medications in general. But when she's thinking of making changes, the psychiatrist needs to be involved.

When Should You Ask for Help?

The short answer is: *Now.* That is, if you've had a comprehensive assessment and you were told you have postpartum depression, then you should ask for help now. If you have determined on your own from reading this book that you are suffering from postpartum depression, you should also ask for help now. However, if you are still not sure that you need help, read the following statements and see if any apply to you:

- I am unable to sleep, even when my baby is sleeping.
- I sometimes think my family would be better off without me.
- I feel overly protective of my baby and I obsessively worry that something bad will happen to her/him.
- I was looking forward to having a baby before I was pregnant, but now I feel like it was a mistake to have a child.
- I do not feel close to my baby.
- I feel as though relationships with my husband, children, or family have deteriorated and I don't know why.
- I feel agitated much of the time and have frequent "meltdowns."
- I feel excessively or inappropriately guilty much of the time.
- I go out of my way to avoid other people.
- I frequently feel like I will never be my old self again.

If even one of these statements applies, you need to get help now.

An Important Sign That You Need Help Now:
Sleep Deprivation

One of the first symptoms you may experience after the birth of your baby is a lack of sleep. While many women may lose sleep due to prolonged labor, the inability to sleep is a warning sign that must be heeded. In fact, one of the ways of predicting the onset of postpartum depression is looking at how much sleep you get in the latter stages of pregnancy, following delivery in the hospital, and during the first several days postpartum.

In terms of treatment, this means that if you *can't* sleep for several hours following the birth of your baby, it's important to ask your doctor for medication to help you get a good night's sleep. Like most women these days, you will probably be in the hospital for 48 hours at the most. It is, therefore, critical that you begin this new journey with as much sleep and support as possible. Remember that everyone is much more likely to become depressed if they can't sleep.

As you recall, not being able to sleep *and* shortened hospital stays due to hospital policies and insurance constraints are risk factors for depression. We recently heard about a hospital that offered an incentive program to women giving birth there. Women considered to be at "low risk" for complications following childbirth were offered one of two rewards if they agreed to go home from the hospital within 24 hours of giving birth. The rewards were either a home visit from a nurse and $200 or the services of a doula in the home for ten hours (we will tell you more about doulas in Chapter 11 when we discuss social support). Such incentive programs, aimed at turning over the hospital population quickly, do not fully appreciate your need for care and the opportunity to recover some lost sleep after giving birth.

As you already know by now, tremendous and rapid hormonal shifts take place in your body when you have a baby. You have just reached a new detour in the hormonal journey that began nine months before, and it's not over yet. Childbirth was a "hairpin curve"! The levels of some of your most important hormones, such as estrogen, progesterone, prolactin, and oxytocin, have just changed dramatically. These hormones have a tremendous effect on sleep, lactation, bonding, and your emotional well-being. Although scientists don't know exactly how and why sleep takes place, they do know that when you are sleep deprived, you experience very serious symptoms.

The longer you stay in the hospital, the more carefully monitored you will be. And if you show signs of postpartum depression, it is hoped that you will begin receiving help before you go home.

Who to Ask for Help

Your obstetrician, nurse, or any physician or psychotherapist who you already trust is a good place to start. If you don't get the help you need, keep speaking out until somebody listens.

You can also ask a friend for a referral to a postpartum depression specialist. More women than you think have been through a similar experience. Most of the women we have treated don't tell their close personal friends that they have postpartum depression in the beginning. A good deal of the time, they learn later that they have friends who have also suffered and kept it a secret. At least one of your friends probably already has the name of a doctor who helped her with postpartum depression.

Don't Delay Treatment

The longer you let depression or anxiety go untreated, the more difficult they are to treat. Furthermore, the longer you experience postpartum depression, the more you and other members of your family will suffer.

Stacy waited thirteen months, and her depression became so severe she was hospitalized. She felt like she had hit bottom. Once she could no longer deny having postpartum depression, she began treatment. By this time, her family was in disarray, and her toddler was showing aggressive behaviors at his preschool. He was also beginning to hit Stacy. With the help of a treatment team and caring professionals, she began to improve and gradually made progress over the next few months.

Elaine started treatment earlier than Stacy did. This was because she recognized her symptoms with her second pregnancy and became proactive in her recovery. "I felt terrible and knew that the depression I had after the birth of my first child was returning," Elaine recalled. "I didn't want to go through that again, nor did I want to put my 2-year-old daughter through the trauma of living with a depressed mom. I phoned my doctor when I recognized the signs of depression."

Our experience as a team is that women who experience moderate to severe postpartum depression get worse without treatment. Treatment is *always* best begun earlier, rather than later. Even at the onset of pregnancy, you may feel symptoms of depression or anxiety, including symptoms of obsessive compulsive disorder. If you begin dealing with the possibility that you are developing postpartum depression, although difficult to confront, you are more likely to have a successful outcome. As with so many other things in life, the better educated and prepared you are, the better your chances of a positive outcome.

8

Medical Treatment
for Postpartum Depression

POINTS TO PONDER IN THIS CHAPTER

- Medical treatment is necessary because your brain chemistry needs to be regulated.
- You may resist taking medication while you are pregnant or breast-feeding.
- Newer medications offer significant advantages in the treatment of postpartum depression.
- If you're not sleeping, that must be corrected with medication.
- Routine use of antidepressants is not as effective with postpartum depression as it is with other depression.

When it's been confirmed through a comprehensive assessment that you have postpartum depression, what kind of treatment do you need?

First and foremost, it is essential that you receive medical treatment. Medical treatment is necessary because your brain chemistry needs to be addressed. Depression of any kind is best treated by a combination of medication and psychotherapy. However, as we've said repeatedly, when it comes to postpartum depression, the most appropriate treatment is a combination of medication, psychotherapy, social support, and parenting advice and training. You could try any one of these approaches by itself, but there is not one approach that will be as effective as all of them together. And sometimes without medication, you won't be able to make use of the other treatments.

Perhaps it's true that not every woman who experiences postpartum depression requires medication. However, most often the key factors in whether or not you will need medication are the current severity and past history of your depression. That is, the longer you've been depressed, and the more severe your symptoms, the more likely you will need medication in order to improve.

If your symptoms are so severe that you are having trouble taking care of yourself and your baby, if you have frequent thoughts about harming your baby (or even harm coming to your baby from other sources), or if you're having suicidal thoughts, then most certainly medication will be the cornerstone of your treatment. However, you may be opposed to taking medication. Like other women we've met, you might give one of these reasons for your reluctance to take medication:

- You think you can get better without medication.
- You think that medications will hurt you.
- You believe in the power of alternative treatment approaches over medications.
- You wish to use only natural herbs or homeopathic remedies.
- You may be concerned about the stigma of taking "psychotropic" medication.
- You may be concerned about the effects of taking medications when you are pregnant or breast-feeding.
- You fear that by taking medication, you will confirm that you're depressed or, even worse, "crazy."
- You are a strong, confident woman who believes you can "tough it out."

You may be like Jessica, an executive in a computer software company. She was used to being in control and successful in her career and personal life. When she became depressed after her son Samuel was born, she was reluctant to take medication. "I've gotten through a lot in my life on sheer willpower and intelligence," she told her therapist, "and I don't think I need medication to beat depression."

Charlene, who came from a large, close family, was diagnosed with postpartum depression three months after her daughter was born. "If I start taking medication," she said, "I'm afraid that my family and friends won't understand. I don't know anyone who takes pills for depression, and I don't want to lose any of my relationships over this."

Julie came in for a consultation with our team because of depression after her twins were born. After listening to our recommendations, she decided on her own to take the popular herb St. John's wort to treat her depression. Within two weeks, she called to say that her symptoms were completely gone and that she was feeling so well she would not need to return to see us. A month later, we were called to meet her in a hospital emergency room because she was having thoughts of harming herself and her babies. Although it was her faith in the power of an herb that may have helped her initially, St. John's wort had no curative effect on these obsessive thoughts. Ultimately, she became much worse.

Natural Herbs and Products Are Not Necessarily Better Than Medications

Aren't natural products and herbs superior to medications? The short answer is not necessarily. You, like many other people, may have some misconceptions about what "natural" means. There are several reasons why natural remedies are not necessarily better than a "manufactured" pill. For one thing, many medications are made from natural products. In pharmacy school we took a course called pharmacognacy. This is simply the study of drugs and medications derived from plants. For example, Metamucil is made from the psyllium (fleawort) seed, Digoxin comes from the foxglove plant (*Digitalis purpurea*), morphine is derived from the poppy plant, and quinine comes from cinchona bark.

Second, just because a substance is "natural" doesn't mean it is good for you. "It's a misconception that anything derived from a plant is better than a synthetic drug," says Dr. Sally Guthrie, an associate professor of pharmacy at the College of Pharmacy and Department of Psychiatry at the University of Michigan. "Many deadly poisons are all natural."

Nicotine and the common, cancer-causing cigarette come from to-bacco plants; vodka is distilled from grain and flavored with juniper berries; and cocaine comes from the coca plant.

One of our patients, Susan, told us she would absolutely not take any prescribed medications for postpartum depression. "I smoke mari-juana," she said, "and that's a *natural* product. It helps to calm me when I'm really anxious."

Like Julie and Susan, you may believe that a "natural" product is safe and effective, and because it is a natural product that you can believe the label. Unfortunately, you can't trust the labels on natural products. "If you take a synthetic medication," Dr. Guthrie says, "at least you know what you're getting and how much of it you're getting." That's not the case with so-called natural herbs and medications.

Herbs are not regulated by the Food and Drug Administration. Be-cause they are not regulated, each product—even individual pills—can (and do) vary in potency. "Buying an herbal product," says Dr. Guthrie, "is a little like buying a bottle of wine. There are good bottles and bad bottles, good years and bad years, and good vineyards and bad vine-yards." And you, as the consumer, have no way of knowing the quality of what you're buying. Furthermore, in a recent study examining the quantity control of capsules in a bottle of 100-mg herbal pills, the cap-sules ranged from 0 mg to 200 mg.

If you're like 75 percent of women in this country, during pregnancy you took some kind of over-the-counter medication. Again, there is the assumption that if a pill is sold over the counter without a prescription, it's going to be safe. This, of course, isn't true.

What is also not true is that refusing to take medication will protect you or your baby if you are seriously depressed. There are far greater risks from untreated depression than there are from taking tested and regulated medications with a proven track record in successfully treating depression. Remember that untreated postpartum depression carries risks not only to a newborn but to the entire family.

Our advice is to keep an open mind about taking medication until you get all the facts and a recommendation from your postpartum depression team. We will tell you in this chapter which medications work well with postpartum depression. But we'll also inform you about the side effects and risks of these medications.

"I got tired of hiding in the closet and feeling so awful," Peggy said when she finally agreed to follow our recommendations about treatment. "I didn't do anything wrong to get postpartum depression, and I don't want to feel guilty anymore. I just want to feel normal again and be able to love and care for my baby."

What Happens in Your Body When You Take Medication

When you take medication to help relieve the symptoms of postpartum depression, the imbalance of neurotransmitters in your body is put back into balance. Because postpartum depression is in part a problem of brain chemistry, you will often require medications to make sure your hormones are functioning smoothly again.

But don't expect medicine to suddenly make you feel happy. Antidepressants don't work that way. One woman said that she expected that taking the antidepressant prescribed by her doctor would be like drinking a martini. "I thought my sadness would quickly go away," she said.

Just as martinis don't cure depression, neither does an antidepressant treat sadness. Antidepressants treat depression. There is a difference between depression and sadness. Depression is a biochemical condition featuring sadness, hopelessness, and guilt. Sadness is a reaction to an external circumstance, is not related to the biochemistry of the brain, and usually goes away on its own.

Because of these differences between sadness and depression, there are differences in treatment. Traditional treatment for major depression involves changing the level of neurotransmitters, and medication for depression often requires several weeks to begin to help you feel less depressed.

The Medications That Work Best with Postpartum Depression

There are many different medications developed and used to treat depression and anxiety. Every person reacts slightly differently to the same medication. Often, finding the right medication or the right combination of medicines will be the result of trial and error by your doctor.

If your physician tries different medications and different dosages, this doesn't mean he doesn't know how to prescribe medications. No doctor can know exactly how you will respond to a medication and which ones will best relieve *your* symptoms. We do know that if you have taken medication for depression or anxiety in the past, that's a good place to start (if your doctor agrees).

Several categories of medications constitute the menu from which most postpartum specialists choose. Some doctors favor just a few of these categories or the medicines within those categories; others favor a wide array of medicines; some use only one at a time; others prefer combinations of medications.

The categories of medicines commonly used in the treatment of postpartum depression include:

- Antidepressants
- Benzodiazepines
- Anticonvulsants
- Atypical Antipsychotics
- Psychostimulants
- Hormones

Although at times we may use medications in all of these categories in treating mood disorders in women, when it comes to treating postpartum depression, our greatest success comes from the use of a combination of antidepressants and atypical antipsychotics. In the past, before atypical antipsychotics were introduced, antidepressants were the treatment of choice. Many physicians, especially obstetricians, still treat postpartum depression as if these newer medications were never developed or made available. Consequently, our approach may be considered novel at times. However, after treating several thousand women with postpartum depression, we've found that success is often achieved by using medications in unique ways.

Often, we find that many physicians are hesitant about prescribing medications for postpartum depression, or they are reluctant to try novel approaches. Our team goes "outside the box" by treating postpartum depression in an aggressive manner because we did not like seeing women, their babies, and their families suffering when their depression was resistant to conventional treatment. We didn't like the pain that women endured when they were wracked by frightening obsessions and debilitating depressions. We didn't like seeing antidepressants increase anxiety before they could lower depression. We also didn't like seeing women riddled with the side effects of medications—and then only experiencing marginal improvement. Our approach, achieved by combining unique medications with psychotherapy, support, and parenting, came about because this treatment approach caused women less pain and suffering in the long run—and it worked.

In the rest of this chapter, the medications we use will be described so you have a better understanding of which medicines you might be prescribed and what you can expect from each.

The Antidepressants

There are four main classes of antidepressant medications used to treat depression. These are the Tricyclics (TCAs), the Selective Serotonin Reuptake Inhibitors (SSRIs) and the Serotonin Norepinephrine Reuptake Inhibitors (SNRIs), and the Monoamine Oxidase Inhibitors (MAOIs).

While there is overlap in the way these four types of antidepressants work, they each work somewhat differently, have different side effects, and may be favored to treat postpartum depression for different reasons. We rarely use MAOIs, and, as you will see in the next few pages, we avoid TCAs and prefer to use the SSRIs and the SNRIs.

The TCAs began to see broad use in treating depression in the early 1950s with the introduction of imipramine (Tofranil), still a popular medication (although not for postpartum depression). The effectiveness of the TCAs was immediately apparent in elevating moods of depressed people, and from the 1960s through the 1980s they were the first line of treatment for major depression.

Although the TCAs are just as effective today in treating depression, obsessive-compulsive disorder (OCD), and panic disorder, their side effects are usually significant, and they are toxic in large doses. Like newer antidepressants (SNRIs), TCAs affect two chemical neurotransmitters, norepinephrine and serotonin, by inhibiting the reuptake process so that these neurotransmitters can carry their messages to other neurons. Neurotransmitters are chemicals that carry messages between nerve cells. The neurotransmitters are secreted by one cell and picked up by receptor proteins on the surface of another. Once the message has been delivered, a neurotransmitter is either destroyed or retrieved into the cell that made it. This process is known as reuptake.

By inhibiting the reuptake of serotonin or norepinephrine, the effects of these neurotransmitters are pronounced.

Some of the most frequently prescribed tricyclics (although not for postpartum depression) are amitriptyline (Elavil), amoxapine (Asendin), clomipramine (Anafranil), desipramine (Norpramin), doxepin (Adapin), imipramine (Tofranil), nortriptyline (Pamelor), protriptyline (Vivactil), and trimipramine (Surmontil).

In practice, we use TCAs infrequently. Most women can't tolerate TCAs at therapeutic doses anyway. In fact, in research studies using tricyclics, most women actually drop out of treatment. Furthermore, TCAs can accumulate in the heart and can cause death in overdose.

In serious postpartum depression, where you might get your days and nights reversed, and your attention, concentration, and memory may be impaired, there is always a potential for an accidental overdose. Further, the side effects of dry mouth, constipation, and urinary retention all are problematic with TCAs (and during the postpartum period you will be more sensitive to urinary retention and constipation). For these reasons, we avoid prescribing TCAs. Instead, we are more apt to prescribe an SSRI or an SNRI.

The selective serotonin reuptake inhibitors (SSRIs) were introduced in the late 1980s and rapidly became the most popular prescribed antidepressants in the United States. The reason why these drugs quickly gained a clinical and popular reputation was because they were effective and safe, and had relatively few side effects. Consequently, they became the drugs of choice for depression, anxiety, and OCD. Like TCAs, most of the SSRIs work by primarily increasing brain levels of the neurotransmitter serotonin, which influences mood, sleep, and appetite. Among the most important SSRIs for the treatment of postpartum depression are citalopram (Celexa), fluoxetine (Prozac), sertraline (Zoloft), and escitalopram oxalate (Lexapro).

These four SSRIs are ones we use in combination with atypical antipsychotics. In fact, all can be effective. The choice of which SSRI we use for a particular person will rest on our experience and best judgment. Often, however, we use fluoxetine (Prozac), in part because it was the first SSRI developed and because it has been the most studied of the SSRIs. Furthermore, it has a long half-life, which means it stays in your body a long time. This can be an advantage for you during postpartum depression because of the propensity (if you're depressed) to miss a dose. When this happens, you are unlikely to experience something that's called discontinuation syndrome. This means that if you abruptly stop a medication or forget to take it, you could experience flu-like symptoms.

Terry, for example, arrived at the hospital with nausea, vomiting, and sweating. A monitor was placed on her abdomen, showing a rapid fetal heart rate. Terry was given fluids, and the fetal heart rate returned to normal. When she was questioned, Terry admitted she had abruptly stopped taking Paxil (an SSRI, which we typically do not use) within the last few days and as a result she and her baby had developed discontinuation syndrome.

Fluoxetine, when compared to other SSRIs, has the largest number of studies in pregnant and breast-feeding mothers. Although articles in the 1980s (such as one that gained a lot of attention in *Time* magazine) suggested that fluoxetine could cause miscarriages and birth defects, more careful analysis of research shows this isn't so.

Prozac has the reputation of increasing anxiety and agitation when started at the therapeutic dose (20 mg). We rarely see this when treating women with postpartum depression, because we start with liquid drops of Prozac at less than 5 mg. In fact, you are likely to respond quite well to 5-mg drops. We then slowly increase the dosage as needed to produce a response. This may take two or more weeks. Prozac is effective in treating most of the symptoms of postpartum depression. Hence the dictum: Start low and go slow.

The SSRIs were developed to be user-friendly. But even though their side effect profile is better, they are not free from side effects—and they don't always work as well as TCAs. SSRIs have equal *response* rates but not equal *remission* rates to the TCAs. Response rate means that there is at least a 50 percent reduction in symptoms. Remission means being completely without symptoms. Remission is the goal of treatment. To increase the remission rates, SNRIs were developed.

SNRIs are Seretonin Norepinephrine Reuptake Inhibitors and are also used to treat depression. Effexor, one of the first SNRIs developed, is a norepinephrine reuptake inhibitor only at higher doses. It may take up to four weeks to get to the higher doses needed for the best response. The newest agent, duloxetine (Cymbalta), is an SNRI at its starting dose. No dosage increases are needed for you to get the full action of this medication. Cymbalta achieves a remission rate similar to the TCAs, but with a better side effect profile than the SSRIs. In clinical trials, it appears to affect women's sexual functioning much less than the SSRIs.

Combinations of Medicines

What has become clear to us after treating a great many women with postpartum depression is that the best recovery rate is obtained with small amounts of two or more medications. Women with postpartum depression tend to be very sensitive to medications and to their side effects. Because of this, we frequently combine a low-dose SSRI and a low-dose atypical antipsychotic. With this combination, we see a more rapid recovery in the symptoms of postpartum depression. And we find success in women whose depression has not responded to other medications or to other forms of treatment.

We do not use antipsychotics because we think you are crazy. In fact, if we thought you were psychotic, you would be on high doses of an antipsychotic. In low doses, these medications boost the antidepressants.

We developed this treatment after working with many women who were resistant to the medications they were taking when referred to us.

Something we observed as interns illustrates our reasoning. This observation had to do with starting an IV on a patient. Often, we, like everyone else—the nurse, the intern, and other first- and second-year interns—had failed to get the IV started. But we noticed that the Chief Resident always got it started. Why was that? Simple. It wasn't because he was more skilled but because he was observant. He didn't try to start the IV in the same places everyone else had tried and failed. That lesson always came back to us as we have learned to treat women with postpartum depression, especially when their depression seemed to resist every effort with medication. We don't keep using medications that don't work. We try something else.

If you're depressed, waiting two to six weeks for a medication to take effect may feel like an eternity. This is too long when you have postpartum depression. Consequently, we augment therapy by adding a medication like olanzapine (Zyprexa) or risperidone (Risperdal). By adding the second medication, we expect that your symptoms will be dramatically improved relatively quickly.

Zoloft is another SSRI we use. Because it often causes sleepiness, this is an advantage if you take Zoloft at night. It doesn't stay in the body as long as Prozac (because it has a shorter half-life). This may be important to some women who may want to stop using antidepressants when pregnant. You can stop taking it when you realize you've missed your first period and may be pregnant. It will be out of your system by the time your baby's circulation is established. Troublesome side effects can include headaches and stomach problems. However, these effects can be minimized or avoided by starting at low doses. It is safe for you to continue taking Zoloft when you are pregnant, and may actually be safer for you and your baby than stopping. Whether you continue or not, though, is a decision that should be made by you, your partner, your obstetrician, and your treatment team.

Citalopram (Celexa) and escitalopram oxalate (Lexapro) are almost chemically identical. They are both effective in treating depression, anxiety, and obsessive compulsive disorder; however, studies show evidence of rapid action but with fewer sexual side effects, especially with Lexapro. Research suggests that babies exposed to Celexa and Lexapro during pregnancy are not adversely affected.

Venlafaxine (Effexor) is the only tested SNRI currently available. It is an SSRI at low doses, and an SNRI at higher doses (of about 225 mg a day). It can cause hypertension at higher doses, but it stays in the body only a short time. If you stop taking it abruptly, however, there is the chance of discontinuation syndrome. The remission rate for depression, especially postpartum depression, is higher than it is with pure SSRIs.

Antipsychotic Medication

When you see the word "antipsychotic," it probably conjures up frightening images. This, of course, may come from associations with the older, typical antipsychotic medications like Thorazine. Drugs like Thorazine were toxic and had irreversible side effects. They, however, were only used in the most seriously ill patients. Today we have newer medications that still share the category "antipsychotic." The differences with these newer medicines are that they are used to treat people who are not nearly as ill, and they are safer. The current generation of antipsychotics are frequently prescribed to help individuals with anxiety, depression, obsessions, and delusions. These new drugs are easier to use and *should be used.*

One of the atypical antipsychotics that we have already mentioned is olanzapine (Zyprexa). We, along with other doctors treating anxiety and depression, use Zyprexa because it is safe and it gets the job done.

Zyprexa is extremely effective for sleep, anxiety, and depression. Its effectiveness has been proven in many studies for the treatment of depression and treatment-resistant depression. Zyprexa has been researched extensively, and when pregnant women took Zyprexa in studies, no birth defects were found. In our own experience with nine pregnant women who took Zyprexa during pregnancy, neither the mothers nor babies were adversely affected. Further, the outcomes for both mothers and babies in these cases, if Zyprexa had not been taken, could have been tragic.

Quetiapine (Seroquel) is an atypical antipsychotic that is effective for treating sleep disorders, anxiety, and depression in higher doses. An advantage of this medication is that it causes less weight gain at lower doses than do other medications. And, like other atypical antipsychotics, there is no indication of any long-term side effects.

Risperidone (Risperdal) is another antipsychotic that has been used as an add-on in the treatment of depression at low doses. It is not sedating, which may be of benefit in women who are sleeping too much, and it doesn't cause weight gain. While it helps to control depression well, it is not effective for anxiety, nor is it recommended when breast-feeding.

Anticonvulsant Medications

We used anticonvulsant medications frequently before the newer antipsychotic medicines were available. Most of the anticonvulsants have the disadvantage of being potentially toxic to the liver and, therefore, requiring blood monitoring. These medications work well, but not as well as the newer antipsychotics. Further, with the newer medications, there is no need for blood testing.

Valproic acid (Depakote) was originally designed to control seizures. It has been found to be very effective in treating anxiety, although by itself it is not useful in treating depression. It is a sedating medication and carries with it a 3 percent risk of spina bifida for your baby if you're taking Depakote during pregnancy. It also tends to increase the risk of cranio-facial abnormalities in newborns. Because of potential interactions with folic acid, we advise that your intake of folic acid be increased during pregnancy when taking Depakote.

Carbamazepine (Tegratol) is an anticonvulsant medication that has been found to be useful to treat anxiety. Like Depakote, it is less effective by itself in the treatment of depression. It has been studied often, particularly in pregnant women, and has about a 1 percent risk of causing neural tube defects. Tegratol tends to lower estrogen levels and may render birth control pills ineffective.

Lamotrigine (Lamictal), another anticonvulsant, has proven to be effective in treating manic depressive illness. Bipolar disorder or manic depressive illness can appear at first as postpartum depression. If you have postpartum depression, an advantage of Lamictal is that it does not appear to increase congenital birth defects. It is not a good medication for anxiety, and a rare side effect is a rash that can progress to Steven's Johnson Syndrome, which can be fatal.

A final anticonvulsant medication that we find helpful in treating the anxiety that accompanies postpartum depression is gabapentin (Neurontin). It does not treat depression, but because it is not addicting, it can be particularly useful in treating anxiety. It also reduces cravings if you have substance abuse problems, and it's frequently used in the treatment of chronic pain.

Benzodiazepines

Benzodiazepines are some of the most potent and effective medications available in treating anxiety. Noted for relieving symptoms in a very short period of time, benzodiazepines can be taken on an "as-needed" basis. While they act rapidly, these medications can cause drowsiness and may lead to dependence and addiction. On the other hand, if you have extreme anxiety or panic attacks, the benzodiazepines will work well in small doses, usually in combination with other, nonaddicting medications.

Benzodiazepines include alprazolam (Xanax), diazepam (Valium), clonazepam (Klonopin), lorazepam (Ativan), zaleplon (Sonata), and zolpidem (Ambien). Valium is not recommended because it lasts an extremely long time in the body and can cause sleepiness. In fact, the benzodiazepines acquired a bad reputation because of Valium, which is not only addicting, but associated with an increase in birth defects such as cleft lip and cleft palate. The newer benzodiazepines, like Xanax, Klonopin, Ativan, Sonata, and Ambien, are highly effective in the treatment of anxiety and are especially good at restoring the sleep-wake cycle that is most often disturbed in women with postpartum depression. Furthermore, these medications have not been shown to increase birth defects. But there are risks to you and your baby. If you use benzodiazepines for a long time, you (and the baby you're carrying) could become dependent on the medicine. If you take these medications while you are pregnant, when your baby is born there will be an abrupt withdrawal of the medication for your baby with the possibility of withdrawal symptoms.

Among the other benzodiazepines, Xanax is a rapid-acting medication that gets in and out of your system quickly and can be effective in reducing panic attacks. Ativan is also good for treating anxiety. It is metabolized differently in your body than the other medications and is less likely to be passed on to your fetus. Klonopin is a long-acting medication, staying in the body a long time. However, although effective in the treatment of anxiety, it has the potential—when taken during pregnancy—to cause respiratory depression in your newborn.

Sonata, which stays in the body a very short time, is used solely for helping you sleep. If you have time constraints (and what new mother doesn't?), it will help you fall asleep, but it will not keep you asleep. You will awaken after no more than an hour or two without feeling drowsy. Sonata can be taken a couple of times a day, especially at night when your baby is sleeping, and you need to rest. Ambien is similar to Sonata, but it stays in your body longer. It causes longer periods of sleep and helps you stay asleep when you don't have time constraints.

Psychostimulants

Our culture is stimulant phobic. Having unreasonable fears that taking a psychostimulant medication will lead to you becoming a "speed freak" or some kind of drug addict is absurd. In our practice, we often use stimulants, which are wonderful medications to augment antidepressants, increase energy, and decrease sleepiness. And not only is it true that women don't become dependent on these medications, but they often use them less often than they should.

When stimulant medicines are used for prescribed purposes, they are safe. In addition, they are especially helpful in the treatment of postpartum depression. We use medications like Adderall, Concerta, and Provigil as augmentation for depression and for women who have attention deficit disorder, sleep disorders, or extreme fatigue.

Adderall (amphetamine-dextroamphetamine) in low doses of 5 to 10 mg is very helpful in elevating your mood rapidly and helping to lift the symptoms of depression. Usually, there is also an easing of the extreme fatigue, lethargy, and need to sleep that accompany depression while taking this medication. Generally, we use Adderall for short periods of time, for instance, eight to twelve weeks.

Methylphenidate (Concerta) is as effective as Adderall in the treatment of sleepiness and lethargy. In our experience, though, Concerta doesn't decrease anxiety, while Adderall does.

Modafinil (Provigil) was developed for use in narcolepsy, or sleeping sickness. We find it very useful as augmentative medication to fight depression itself, as well as the fatigue and lethargy associated with postpartum depression. In our experience, it has little potential for causing dependence; however, it may cause headaches.

Hormones

The final type of medication we use in treatment is hormones. The Estrodial patch, for instance, decreases the symptoms of depression when combined with an antidepressant. Progesterone, on the other hand, is a hormone we rarely prescribe, as it has been shown to be relatively ineffective, while sometimes actually increasing depression.

Breast-feeding

You may be concerned about taking medication while you are breast-feeding. While this is a very normal concern, medications for depression and anxiety are frequently prescribed to breast-feeding women these days. You may be relieved to know that the use of antidepressants during breast-feeding has been studied, and the results are encouraging.[1] Based on a thorough review of the many studies related to the use of medication during breast-feeding, we strongly recommend that you continue to take your prescribed medication and breast-feed your baby if you:

- have suicidal thoughts or thoughts of harming your baby;
- fear being alone with your baby;
- have delusions or hallucinations;
- have difficulty functioning on a daily basis;
- are not responsive to supportive or psychological therapy alone.

The benefits of taking medication under these circumstances will almost always outweigh the risks of exposing your infant to medication. If you stop breast-feeding while you are taking medication, then your baby and you will both lose out.

Earlier in this chapter, we provided you with considerable information about the medications used by postpartum depression specialists. As we indicated, with some of the medications there are potentially dangerous side effects when pregnant or breast-feeding. But whether you breast-feed or not, taking medication should always be discussed with your partner, your pediatrician, and your prescribing psychiatrist or psychopharmacologist. In all cases, you need to weigh the risks and benefits of both breast-feeding and taking medication. Keep these facts in mind:

- The risk of tobacco in breast milk is much higher than that of psychotropic medications in breast milk.

- The risk of your untreated depression or anxiety is often considerably higher than the risk of breast-feeding on medications.
- Ninety-five percent of breast-feeding mothers take at least one medication during the first postpartum week, 17 to 25 percent take medications in the two weeks surrounding their fourth postpartum month, and up to 5 percent will take at least one medication throughout the entire breast-feeding period.[2]

Researchers and physicians are inclined toward great caution when advising nursing mothers about taking medication. While caution is important, we are not quite as concerned with the postpartum use of medications. Instead, we are greatly concerned about serious and long-lasting dangers for both your bond with your baby and your baby's development if you choose to remain depressed and anxious rather than risk taking medication.

Most medications will pass through your system and into your breast milk, but usually only in very tiny amounts. Although a *very few* of these medications could potentially cause a problem for your baby, this is not the case for the vast majority of medications you are likely to be prescribed for postpartum depression.

If you have concerns about the effect of a medication on your baby, ask your physician. If you decide that the risks are too great, ask about an alternative medication that may be more acceptable during breast-feeding. Most medications we prescribe do not appear to have long-term effects for your baby, and any adverse effects are usually reversible when you stop taking the medication or when you stop breast-feeding.

Your postpartum team, along with your pediatrician, should monitor you and your baby while you are taking medication. If you should see a change in your baby's behavior, like colic, irritability, or disrupted sleep patterns while you are taking medication and nursing, you should tell your pediatrician and your team. Although we can't tell you that every medication is completely "safe or harmless" for your baby, neither can we tell you that your baby is completely safe from harm if you are anxious or depressed.

Approximately 50 percent of new mothers will begin breast-feeding in the hospital.[3] Following World War II, about 20 percent of mothers breast-fed. In the 1960s through the 1980s, 60 percent of mothers breast-fed,[4] and since the 1980s, there has been a slight decline in the numbers of mothers who breast-feed.

We are not sure why there has been a decline in the popularity of breast-feeding. Some of the reasons may be the inaccessibility of lactation consultants and other professionals who can assist you if you want to breast-feed your baby.

Cindy, for example, tried to breast-feed her new baby in the hospital. Her insurance didn't cover a lactation consultant, her doctor told her to ask the nurses for help, and the nurses were busy and unavailable. In fact, Cindy learned that the term used in hospitals by nurses for breast-feeding is "ramming." That's just how Cindy said she felt when her baby was literally thrown on her chest by the nurse. Her nursing lasted exactly three days. By that time, her nipples were cracked and bleeding, and her spirit wasn't far behind. "I felt like I failed at one of my first major jobs as a mother," Cindy said.

The policies of some hospitals discourage breast-feeding by mandating supplemental feeding and also by "pushing" commercially prepared formula discharge packs.[5] Furthermore, early discharge from hospitals and increased marketing of formulas, along with work environments that are unfriendly to breast-feeding, may also contribute to the belief that it's better to avoid breast-feeding.

However, you should be aware that the U.S. Department of Health and Human Services, the American Academy of Pediatrics, the American College of Obstetrics and Gynecology, and the American Academy of Family Physicians all recommend breast-feeding. Breast-fed infants benefit through having:

- lower rates of hospital admissions and illness in general
- lower ear, respiratory, urinary, and intestinal tract infections
- less eczema and fewer food allergies
- increased ease in digestion
- possible protection against Type I diabetes
- stronger immune systems throughout life
- higher IQs when tested at age 7 or 8

And mothers who breast-feed have:

- quicker weight loss and
- protection against certain cancers, including breast and ovarian

Studies show that spending time with your baby right from the start will help you feel more confident as a mother. It gives you precious time with your baby, helps you to feel competent, especially if you are depressed, and is likely to increase your sense of attachment to your baby. Also, when you're nursing, your body produces oxytocin, a hormone that helps protect you against postpartum bleeding. Many breast-feeding mothers also find it easier compared to the repetitive chore of heating formula and preparing seemingly endless bottles at all times of the day and night. Last, but by no means least, there is a financial benefit to breast-feeding. It is far less expensive than buying formula.

But what if you don't want to breast-feed?

"I felt tremendous pressure to breast-feed," Monica said. "Everyone told me I had to breast-feed because it's healthier and better. So I did nurse my baby. But I wasn't happy about it, and soon I stopped."

"They kept pushing that cart at me, telling me I had to breast-feed," Sandy said tearfully. "I was pushing it right back, saying, 'I can't.'"

"My biggest worry of all during the last month of my pregnancy was the thought of breast-feeding," Miriam explained. "I was very uncomfortable with it because it felt sexual. But other people told me I had a duty to give my baby the best nutrients. Then, I felt there was no way to get out of it."

After she gave birth to her daughter, Miriam was pressured by a nurse who told her, "You'll do fine, Honey, it's easy." Miriam was further embarrassed when the nurse "yanked up my hospital gown, exposing me to everyone in the hallway." Miriam begged the nurse to feed her baby for her. "You've got to do this," the nurse replied. "This is your job."

Breast-feeding isn't for everyone. If you breast-feed to please others, you only increase the stress in your life. That stress may be increased by confusion and conflict. For instance, Kara was confused about what to do when she was diagnosed with postpartum depression and was prescribed medication at the same time.

"After my son was born, I began to breast-feed him," Kara said. "He had problems latching on, and the sleep deprivation was taking a toll on me. I fed him every two or three hours, but I feel like I wasn't bonding much with him because my mind was thinking more about getting enough sleep, so I could function during the day."

After she was diagnosed with postpartum depression, a doctor advised Kara to stop breast-feeding. "I thought breast-feeding was the right thing to do, and then I was told not to," Kara said. "I didn't know what was right."

What's right is what is right for you and for your baby. That's a decision that you, or you and your partner, can make. However, when it comes to choosing the right medications for you, it will depend on your treatment team and your doctor. The factors that will likely be taken into consideration will include:

- the symptoms and severity of your postpartum depression
- past medication treatment you've had and how you responded to it
- your ability to function in day-to-day tasks

- your psychological history and the current risk of harm to yourself or your baby
- the age and health of your baby

If you have taken medications for depression before, let your doctor know what they were and how you responded. If possible, you want to use the medications that were effective previously. This is not the time to experiment with new treatments.

You may also have anxiety or obsessive thoughts that if you breast-feed, your baby won't get enough to eat. Some depressed mothers worry about this because they can't see or measure what the baby is getting. If that sounds like you, remember that if your baby appears satisfied and is gaining weight, she's probably getting plenty to eat. Your newborn's stomach is roughly the size of a marble. At ten days of age, her stomach has grown to the size of a shooter marble, and at three months of age it's the size of a golf ball. She doesn't need a five-course meal! But it is important to pay attention to how she behaves when nursing, how she latches on, and whether she seems content when she is finished. Your baby has to learn how to nurse, just like you do.

Medications and Breast-feeding

Studies show that taking the SSRIs, TCAs, and the short-acting benzodiazepines while breast-feeding appear relatively safe. If you're taking lithium for manic depression, however, you should not breast-feed. And the long-term risks of certain antipsychotics, especially in high doses, are not yet clear.[6]

The antidepressants, both the TCAs and the SSRIs, are the medications we have the most information on. For instance, we know that if you are taking an SSRI or a TCA during pregnancy, there is no increased risk of birth defects. We know that when you're breast-feeding, the baby will receive some fraction of the dose you're taking. There is no reason to believe that trace amounts of medication in a newborn have a greater effect than the high doses experienced during pregnancy, and clinical observations confirm this.

No matter what medication you've been prescribed, we recommend that your postpartum team monitor the health of both you and your baby. Whenever you note changes in your baby's behavior when you are taking medication and nursing, be sure to tell your pediatrician. While we can never completely reassure you about the safety of every medication, we think that you are at your best when you are depression-free. Your baby will be, too.

There are many reasons to breast-feed, and we believe in encouraging breast-feeding unless there are data that show clear risk to the newborn. This means that with some of the newer medications for which we have limited data, we tell women the risk is unknown to the newborn, but we know there are many benefits of breast-feeding for the newborn. Antidepressants in general have not been found to cause harm. The risk–benefit ratio clearly sits on the side of benefit.

Francine, who had severe postpartum depression, was taking Zyprexa and Prozac throughout her pregnancy and she had a strong desire to breast-feed. When given information about the medications that were helping her, she was not entirely reassured. But having weighed the risks and benefits to herself and the newborn, she decided to breast-feed.

This was almost fifteen months ago. Now, Francine's son, who is 18 months of age, has attained all of the normal developmental milestones.

Psychological Treatment for Postpartum Depression

- Psychotherapy is a necessary ingredient of your treatment plan.
- Cognitive-behavioral and interpersonal therapies can be effective in treating postpartum depression.
- You may find the support of group therapy helpful.
- Individual, group, and family therapies may be recommended for you.

Psychotherapy is not just an optional ingredient in the treatment of postpartum depression. It is a necessity—particularly if you want the best and the most expedient recovery. Don't just take our word for it. There is research to back this up.

- A study of depressed people reported in 2000 in the *British Medical Journal* found that depressed patients who receive cognitive-behavioral therapy or counseling improve significantly more than other patients who are treated only with medication by a physician.[1]
- The *Archives of General Psychiatry* reported recently that in a study of 120 women suffering from postpartum depression that

interpersonal counseling is effective in reducing the symptoms of postpartum depression.[2]

Medication alone is often effective. Psychotherapy alone is frequently helpful for mild to moderate depression but not for severe depression. With the combination of medication and psychotherapy, you significantly raise the chance that you're going to get better sooner, and that your recovery will be longer-lasting.

If you have moderate to severe postpartum depression, you may feel like you've lost control of your life. Or that it isn't your life at all. On the other hand, you may feel as if there is no hope that you will ever have the life you've planned.

You will be encouraged to take the recommendations of your treatment team and enter psychotherapy. Because depression is more than a chemical imbalance, particularly postpartum depression, there are issues that should be addressed in counseling, even when you are taking medication. Often, though, you must become stable on medications before you can benefit from psychotherapy.

Why is psychotherapy critical now, and why is it so different from what we usually think of as therapy?

"I'll take the pills, but I don't have time to sit around and talk about my life," Alicia said when she begrudgingly went for her first appointment with a psychologist. "It just makes me cry. Maybe if I don't talk about it, it will go away. Besides, I don't have time to shower, and I'm already seeing a psychiatrist. When am I supposed to do therapy?"

You may feel like Alicia. You probably just want to stop feeling depressed and get on with your life and your new family. We can understand why you might feel this way. Yet the psychologist or counselor, as part of your treatment team, plays an important role. Your therapist, as we said in Chapter 7, is the quarterback who coordinates the team and communicates the signals to the other team players. You need someone who is an expert in postpartum depression and is also able to provide guidance to you and your family while coordinating treatment.

Choosing Your Psychotherapist

Who should be your psychotherapist? The gender of your therapist doesn't matter, unless it matters to you. It also doesn't matter whether he or she has a master's degree or a doctorate, whether it's in psychology, social work, guidance and counseling, or nursing. What *is* important is that your therapist is trained, experienced, and specializes in postpartum depression. It is also important that he or she is part of a treatment team that will include a psychiatrist or psychopharmacologist who specializes in postpartum depression.

The members of your treatment team should possess certain important qualities, including experience and maturity. They will, in other words, be "seasoned." It's in your best interest to make sure that the members of your treatment team are not fresh out of school. Although everyone needs to start somewhere, don't let him or her start on you when you have postpartum depression. On one hand, you don't want someone treating you who might panic and put you in the hospital if you mention that you have some of the less understood symptoms of postpartum depression—like obsessive compulsive disorder or delusions. On the other hand, you need to be able to trust that when you are honest with your feelings, your psychotherapist knows when it *is* time for hospitalization.

Individual Therapy

Talk therapy helps. Research indicates three things about talk therapy: (1) You are likely to benefit from seeing a therapist whom you perceive as warm and caring; (2) You will get more from a therapist with whom you can identify and whom you strive to emulate; and (3) Your depression will improve by you having a therapist who uses a cognitive-behavioral or interpersonal approach.

Notice that we did not say that you will get help for your depression by a psychoanalytic approach or by analyzing how you got depressed. Psychoanalytically oriented therapies are wonderful, but they don't lend themselves to the treatment of postpartum depression. They require a long-term process that could take years. You have a baby to raise, and you cannot afford to wait several years to stop feeling depressed. Cognitive therapies are based on the premise that changes in values, beliefs, and attitudes will lead to changes in thinking and in behavior. In cognitive-oriented therapy, the therapist focuses on distortions in thinking. You may feel inadequate or incompetent as a mother. Your therapist can help you correct this. By eliminating distortions in your thinking, you will feel less anxious and depressed, and your coping skills will improve.

Talk therapy can be very practical at times. We believe that a major purpose of talk therapy is to decrease anxiety. For instance, Sondra, who entered treatment after being diagnosed with severe postpartum depression, needed help to relieve her anxiety related to her baby. "Justin stops breathing at times, and my mother gets extremely upset when it happens," Sondra said. "Obviously, I do, too, but Justin's pediatrician said not to worry about it."

Sondra's therapist told her and her husband that a local hospital had a sleep apnea department set up just to evaluate that kind of problem. The therapist helped these new parents arrange with the hospital for Justin to have an evaluation. During the first visit, a 24-hour monitor was placed on Justin, and the staff explained to Sondra that the monitor would help them make a diagnosis. Sondra learned that Justin had reflux and not apnea. "The doctor at the hospital told me exactly what to do when Justin holds his breath," Sondra said. "I also felt as though the weight of the world had been lifted off my shoulders. I felt like the pediatrician had dismissed my concerns, but I was afraid to say anything. After all, he's the doctor."

A therapist should be oriented toward problem solving. When you have postpartum depression, it's not always the time to tell your entire life story. When you're feeling more stable, you may want to gain some insight into your background and current relationships. In the meantime, it's important to focus on those things that will restore you to a daily level of functioning like you had before you were depressed.

During individual talk therapy, we focus on important practical problems that need more immediate attention. These may include:

- How you're sleeping.
- The positive role of exercise when you're up to it, starting with brief walks.
- What your diet is like and whether you're eating enough to sustain you.
- How much stress you feel and how you're coping with your stress.
- How you're dealing with any recent traumas or the triggering of any past traumas.
- Setting goals and establishing priorities.
- Developing routines and providing needed structure in your life.
- Managing your fears.
- Creating or accessing your social support system.
- Decreasing perfectionism and developing realistic expectations.
- Educating you about postpartum depression and the biological aspects of the disorder.
- Reassuring you that you're not crazy.

Your therapist can—and will—talk to you about many issues and concerns in your life. But don't be surprised when one of those issues is how you're taking care of yourself. Your lifestyle can be an issue. If you're not eating or getting enough sleep, if you are engaging in self-defeating behaviors (such as smoking or using drugs or alcohol), or if you aren't exercising, your therapist will explore these issues with you and guide you in your recovery.

We have good evidence these days that anxiety, depression, and stress can all be reduced or protected against by exercise.[3] In addition, studies of people experiencing major depression show that daily aerobic exercise can substantially improve your mood in a short period of time. Consequently, your therapist should encourage you to exercise, even though you may not feel like doing so or lack the motivation and self-discipline. That's where group therapy or a support group can help.

Group Therapy

Group therapy and social support groups can provide many benefits for you when you are depressed. Just finding out that you're not alone in what you've been thinking and feeling has tremendous value for many women with postpartum depression.

"When I first went to group therapy," Teresa said, "I heard other women saying what I had been feeling and was afraid to say out loud. It was a relief to know I wasn't crazy."

Groups can be supportive, and often the women in them are able to come up with many positive ways to help each other. For example, it is frequently helpful to hear how others have gotten their husbands to be more supportive, and it is helpful to receive suggestions from other women about what to tell your friends and your family about your illness. One of the things we have found when women absolutely won't talk about being diagnosed with postpartum depression is that if they say they have a sleep disorder, they get less criticism and more help. Since not being able to sleep is a frequent symptom in postpartum depression, some women would rather talk about this aspect of their illness.

Furthermore, the encouragement and support you get from others to stay on your medication, to exercise, and to eat properly can be invaluable as you put forth efforts to get back on your feet. Ongoing social support can be most important when you may have few other positive and encouraging resources in your life.

We have found that closed-end groups work best when you have postpartum depression. A closed-end group means that it meets for a set number of weeks, for example, six weeks. Open-ended groups, in which women come and go over a long period of time, don't work as well because "old members" may talk about relapses or get emotionally and personally stuck. This can be discouraging for you if you're just entering the group. Additionally, if women have made remarkable progress, newer members may feel out of place and awkward when they tell how they're feeling at the beginning of their treatment.

We may suggest you limit your therapy, at least temporarily, to individual therapy if you have obsessive thoughts or compulsive behaviors. Being obsessive, you may begin to take on the symptoms and worries of others in the group when they talk about their own thoughts, feelings, and problems. Also, if you're so sensitive that you feel badly for others, this may interfere with your own recovery. When that is likely, individual therapy may be the best option.

Group therapy sessions should be an opportunity for women at about the same place in their recoveries to learn and support each other. This happens best in a short-term group that provides education and structure.

Similarly, if you were diagnosed with depression while still pregnant, you will do better in a group of pregnant women—rather than one made up largely of women who have already delivered their babies. If you are pregnant, you have a unique set of problems and should not be exposed to problems that you don't have. You might begin to worry more and feel like you are never going to get better.

We discourage women in group therapy from socializing outside of group while in therapy. It's not that you don't need to increase your social network. However, remember that your primary goal is to receive help and support. When you socialize outside of the group, you may shift your focus to helping each other—ordinarily not a bad thing—at a time when you need to concentrate on your own recovery.

We do encourage you to bring family members with you to group therapy. It is not uncommon in our family groups for women to bring their sisters, mothers, or husbands.

"I wanted everyone to know what a wonderful mother and sister I have," Rebecca said in group therapy one evening. "So I brought them with me so you all could meet them. I wouldn't be getting better if it wasn't for them."

Having family members attend group shows their support for you and can often be helpful in encouraging you to reach out for support from your family.

Marital Therapy

Marital therapy might sound like a good idea if you're having conflicts with your partner. However, we don't feel that marital therapy is *ever appropriate* when postpartum depression is present until after the depression has been treated successfully. Marital therapy is stressful and may only increase the conflict between you and your partner. It may also bring new stressors (such as consideration of separation or divorce) at a time when you should be working to reduce stress and increase your coping skills.

Marital therapy should be reserved for a time when both you and your partner are healthy enough to look at yourselves and make changes in your relationship. After your postpartum depression has been conquered, you and your partner can resolve any remaining conflicts.

Until then, here are some steps to take to improve your relationship:

- Listen to your partner.
- Avoid distractions and talk face-to-face without television, music, or a crying baby.

- Focus on the problem at hand. Make sure each of you fully understands the other's point of view before trying to solve the problem.
- Stay on one issue. Don't drag other problems or past behaviors into the discussion.
- Reserve the right to take a break and to stop the conversation if it gets ugly.
- Deal with the obstacles. If one of you is unwilling to talk, ask why.

We often are told of a conflict between partners about sex when postpartum depression is present. Generally, women are not interested in sex during the three months following the birth of a child. When postpartum depression is present, this period of time can go on much longer. Depression reduces sex drive, feeling bad about body image decreases sex drive, fatigue reduces sex drive, and some medications can reduce sex drive. What we can tell you is that if you had a good sexual relationship before you had a baby, just be patient and don't try to fix it and create a bigger problem. The best predictor of behavior is past behavior. Just give it time.

Family Therapy

Family therapy is often appropriate and recommended in the treatment of postpartum depression. Postpartum depression is rough on the whole family, even extended family members like your parents, your husband's parents, your siblings, and, of course, your older children.

Your partner or family members may experience a range of emotions including shame, embarrassment, fear, anger, and guilt related to your depression. You may feel that you're neglecting others in your family because of your depression. The support network you have in your family may well be strained (it usually is when postpartum depression exists) because you have your hands full just trying to function on a daily basis and because you may be isolating yourself at this time.

At first, everyone was sympathetic and understanding of Sylvia's depression. "But the longer I was depressed," Sylvia said in group therapy, "the more distant and less sympathetic everyone was. They thought I should be better and they couldn't understand why I couldn't host our usual gala Thanksgiving Day party. They thought I was mad at them. The truth was, they were mad at me for being depressed."

In family therapy, attended by Sylvia and her husband, her children, and in-laws, everyone got a chance to express their feelings and concerns. "We all ended up crying and saying how much we missed her," Sylvia's husband said. "We all had a chance to tell her that we were there for her and that we still loved her."

It's easy to see how postpartum depression can stress out even the most loving family and the strongest marriage. You and your husband or partner may disagree or argue over discipline of the children, or you may have difficulty finding time for each other because you may be exhausted from caring for your baby or even trying to care for yourself. Family therapy can be very useful in addressing these issues.

Although there are various types of family therapy—just as there are different types of group and individual therapies—all have the same goals of strengthening the family as a system and improving the ability of all family members to communicate better and solve problems more effectively.

Substance Abuse

Prenatal exposure to alcohol is one of the leading preventable causes of birth defects, mental retardation, and neurological disorders in the United States.[4] Between 1991 and 1995, alcohol use by pregnant women increased substantially, and alcohol use by nonpregnant women of childbearing age increased slightly.[5] Substance abuse in pregnant women and mothers frequently goes unrecognized because women themselves don't admit they are abusing alcohol or drugs. They often say, "I'm just using it."

Alcohol use and illicit drug use can markedly alter medications, and at times render them totally ineffective.

Elaine had a history of alcoholism, although she remained abstinent through her pregnancy. After the delivery of a healthy baby boy and upon discharge from the hospital, she began to drink alcohol heavily. "I don't know why I was able to control my drinking during my pregnancy," Elaine said after she started treatment for alcoholism, "but give in to it after my baby was born. You'd think I'd be so happy that I wouldn't have to drink."

Just as the hormonal changes of childbirth affect other things for you, so will those changes affect the course of your recovery from alcoholism or other drug use. We know that a majority of women relapse in alcohol and drug addiction premenstrually, and this is because of the rapid hormonal fluctuation. The same thing happens right after you give birth to your baby.

Alcohol is a toxin, and the more you drink, the more toxic it is. It is also a central nervous system depressant, and to avoid serious consequences for both you and your baby, alcoholism (and other addictions) requires its own specific kind of treatment.

Eating Disorders

The more we work with women suffering with postpartum depression, the more we are aware that many women have eating disorders. An eating disorder can include binge eating, anorexia, and bulimia before you are pregnant, and these same types of disorders only seem to get worse during pregnancy. However, for some, eating disorders develop for the first time only after you give birth.

It is especially true that you can develop an eating disorder after your baby is born if you experienced a very stressful or traumatic labor or delivery. An eating disorder will dramatically exacerbate your depression and make it more difficult for you to respond to the treatment you're getting. If you hide your eating problem, treatment of you as a whole person becomes impossible.

A hurdle to you admitting that you have an eating disorder may be that the disorder has "worked" for you. That is, you may be reluctant to admit that food is a problem needing treatment if you've been "successful" at keeping your weight under control by purging or starving yourself. Of course, like substance abuse, you will need specialized help in order to have your eating disorder treated appropriately.

Attention Deficit Disorder and Attention Deficit Hyperactivity Disorder

Attention Deficit Disorder (ADD) is more common in women than Attention Deficit Hyperactivity Disorder (ADHD); however, both forms of this disorder include difficulties with sustained concentration and attention.

When you have both ADD and depression, it makes treatment much more difficult. As with children with ADD or ADHD, you as an adult will not benefit nearly as much from psychotherapy as you will from medication. And, both ADD and ADHD can be treated successfully with psychostimulant medication.

Although there is some potential for you to become addicted to the traditional psychostimulants, such as Ritalin and Adderall, a new medication is now available to treat ADD. Atomoxetine (Strattera) was recently approved for use with ADD and ADHD. Women who take Strattera note improved memory and attentiveness, and they report that it decreases the fatigue and lethargy that often goes along with postpartum depression—without causing sleep problems at night. Because Strattera is not addicting there is clearly an advantage for you if you have a substance abuse problem.

Hospitalization

Sometimes, when your postpartum depression (or substance abuse or eating disorder) is so severe, hospitalization may be an option. This was true for Marisa.

"I waited so long to ask for help for my depression," Marisa said, "that my husband finally took me to an emergency room. I was admitted to the psychiatric ward and stayed for three days."

By that point, Marisa was drained of all her energy, and was severely depressed. "I hadn't eaten or showered in several days," she later said, "and I hadn't slept in three or four days. Basically, I just wanted to die."

When she was stabilized and came home, she had a different view of her experience than she had at first—when she was frightened about being in a psychiatric ward. "When my husband took me to the hospital," she said, "I had no idea I would be on a psychiatric unit, and at first, it was quite unnerving. Looking back now, it was the best thing that could have happened. They gave me medication as soon as I got there and I think I slept for about twelve hours."

The next day, her husband brought her clothes and shampoo. Marisa took a shower, and that made her feel better. "The medication they gave me seemed to work instantly," Marisa said, "and within two days, I began to feel much better."

It is possible that there may be times when you and your therapist discuss hospitalization. There are two things that hospitalization can do for you if you have severe postpartum depression. First, it can provide a place for you to go to be safe until you are able to care appropriately for yourself and your baby. Second, it is a place where you can go to have your medications adjusted much more quickly than can happen on an outpatient basis. In the hospital, you will be monitored 24 hours a day.

Following hospitalization, day hospital or day treatment is often a good transition back to being at home. In day treatment, you will go to the hospital for the day and return home at night. You will see a member of your team on a daily basis, and you will participate in both individual and group psychotherapies—probably every day.

We are not aware of any inpatient or outpatient hospital programs in the country at this time that offer separate treatment for groups of women with postpartum depression. You may see this as a positive sign, although you may think that being hospitalized and in groups with both men and women and a range of many other psychiatric diagnoses can be further traumatic.

It doesn't promote bonding when a psychiatric floor doesn't allow you to see your baby. Although we understand that hospitals are not the best places for babies, we believe that even when hospitalization is in your best interest, keeping you and your baby apart is not. However, change is occurring.

Recently, our team hospitalized a woman who was breast-feeding her baby. The hospital was extremely helpful and offered to assist Cynthia with a breast pump so that her baby could still have her breast milk. They also offered to send a pediatrician down to the emergency room to instruct Cynthia's husband in how to transition their son to formula, if that's what they chose to do. When Cynthia left the hospital after three days, she was on medication, sleeping, less depressed, and able to resume breast-feeding. She also did the appropriate thing by scheduling an appointment with her therapist and her psychiatrist before leaving the hospital.

Alternative Treatment for Postpartum Depression

POINTS TO PONDER IN THIS CHAPTER

- One-third of U.S. health care dollars are spent on various herbs and alternative medications.
- Prayer is the most commonly used form of alternative medicine.
- Herbs can be dangerous during pregnancy.
- Herbs are not effective in moderate to severe postpartum depression.
- Other forms of alternative medicine can effectively complement traditional treatment.
- If you are using an alternative treatment, you should tell your physician.

Are we making progress in medicine—or regressing? Here is one way of looking at the history of medicine:

- 2000 B.C.: Here, eat this root.
- A.D. 2000: That root is heathen. Say this prayer.
- 1850: That prayer is superstition. Drink this potion.
- 1940: That potion is snake oil. Swallow this pill.

- 1985: That pill is ineffective. Take this antibiotic.
- 2003: That antibiotic is artificial. Eat this root.

In effect, that's about the way we've progressed in the last 4000 years—starting with roots and ending with roots.[1] As far as the treatment of postpartum depression is concerned, we hope that we are not regressing in medical treatment and that we are using some of the modern advantages of science and technology. However, what concerns us the most is that you are treated effectively.

In this chapter, we will tell you what we consider to be good alternative medicine, and how alternative medicines and therapies may have an impact on you during pregnancy, childbirth, and after your baby arrives. We will share the best evidence we have, along with our clinical experience and common sense.

We have learned that what is defined as complementary alternative medicine depends on where you live in the world, which side of the stethoscope you're on, and what year it is. The term "alternative medicine" brings with it many different opinions and emotions. In general, *alternative* implies that it is "other than" the norm, the traditional, the accepted, or commonly practiced. The term *complementary* implies that it is "in addition" to something else. Using just the term *alternative* may be inaccurate in referring to a host of less traditional treatments. Therefore, we will use the broader term complementary alternative medicine.

First, here are some astounding statistics:

- In the United States today, 30 to 40 percent of people use some kind of unconventional practices in any one year. In Asia and other parts of the world, the numbers are higher.
- From 1990 to 1997, the number of visits to alternative practitioners went from 427 million to 629 million per year in this country. This was considerably more visits than to all primary care practitioners in those same years.[2]

- The amount of money paid out-of-pocket during those same years rose from $10 billion to $27 billion. This is about the same as what is spent on conventional care, and more than what is spent on hospital care.
- An estimated one-third of the health care dollars in the United States are going to stores and shops for alternative medicines.

So, what are the various complementary alternative medicines that are garnering so much attention and so much money? Here is a sampling of approaches for treating postpartum depression:

Prayer and spiritual healing
Herbal medicine
Homeopathy
Naturopathy
Nutrition
Light therapy
Transcendental meditation (TM)
Biofeedback
Hypnosis
Yoga/hatha yoga/tai chi
Massage therapy
Acupuncture
Exercise
Pet therapy

Complementary Alternative Therapies We Endorse

Prayer and Spiritual Healing

You might not view prayer and spiritual healing as a form of alternative medicine, but according to some people spiritual help and guidance is the most common complementary alternative medicine approach used in this country.[3] And even the conservative *Wall Street Journal* devoted a major article on the scientific studies of prayer.[4] Surveys report that 75 percent of patients believe that physicians should address spiritual issues *for* and *with* them.

One-third of medical schools in the United States have now developed courses in alternative or complementary medicine, which address spiritual issues and prayer.[5] David B. Larson, M.D., a former researcher at the National Institute of Mental Health, said that when he was in medical school, his professors taught him that religion is actually *harmful* to the ill. On the contrary, research shows that religion is highly beneficial in preventing both mental and physical illness.

Going to religious services or praying regularly may prevent illness and help you cope more effectively with both stress and disease. We think it can be a useful approach for you to add to your treatment for postpartum depression.

Nutrition

Nutrition is extremely important during all stages in life. During pregnancy, it is even more critical. Nutritional counseling may be very helpful, especially during pregnancy and when you are experiencing postpartum depression. During these times, your nutrition is important and nutritional advice can be valuable in helping you counteract some side effects of certain medications, including weight gain.

Light Therapy

Light therapy involves being exposed to strong indoor light. It can be beneficial for the treatment of seasonal affective disorder (SAD), which often occurs during winter months in some high-latitude locations. Always consult with your physician before using any alternative therapy during pregnancy, including light therapy. Light therapy may be helpful in complementing other treatments for postpartum depression. It is not sufficient by itself to treat moderate to severe postpartum depression.

Transcendental Meditation

Transcendental meditation is a combination of a sense of serenity and a connection with a greater power. In the 1970s, Dr. Herbert Benson, a specialist in cardiovascular medicine at Harvard Medical School, determined that transcendental meditation and various relaxation techniques are similar. Meditation and relaxation approaches can lower your heart rate and improve your blood pressure, while reducing your stress. We would encourage you to use any accepted form of meditation or relaxation when you're being treated for postpartum depression.

Biofeedback

Biofeedback, which involves learning to regulate your autonomic responses to stress and anxiety, has significant positive effects on pain control. When trained in biofeedback, you can learn to slow your heart rate and reduce your anxious responses, which can be very important in dealing with your postpartum depression.

Yoga, Hatha Yoga, and Tai Chi

Yoga, hatha yoga, and tai chi all tend to increase positive energy through bodily movement. They are helpful for dealing with stress and can increase optimism and self-confidence. We encourage you to engage in yoga or tai chi, particularly in the later stages of postpartum depression treatment. Since these approaches to treatment involve physical movement, make sure you check with your doctor before beginning these programs during pregnancy.

Massage Therapy

Massage therapy is extremely valuable as a stress reliever. However, *make sure you check with your doctor, and make sure that you let your massage therapist know you are pregnant.* Pressure on the wrists and the ankles can stimulate the uterus, which you don't want when you are pregnant. There is such a thing as "prenatal massage," and this is recommended over a standard massage. If you are depressed, massage is very valuable as it can help you relax because the power of touch is healing. You may not be ready for touching by your partner, as you may fear it will lead to sex. A massage from a skilled massage therapist may, therefore, be safer until you are less depressed and ready for more physical interaction with your partner.

Exercise

Exercise is a complementary alternative medicine that we can heartily recommend. If you have been exercising regularly prior to pregnancy, you should continue throughout your pregnancy. While exercise promotes a wonderful lifestyle in general, when you are depressed or anxious, you may not be able to exercise regularly. When you're ready, your postpartum team will recommend exercise for all of the reasons that you already know.

Pet Therapy

Don't underestimate the value of having a pet. It has been found that having a pet at home is sometimes just as valuable as support from a spouse or your family.[6]

Complementary Alternative Therapies We Do *Not* Endorse

Herbal Medicine

The World Health Organization reports that approximately 80 percent of the 4 billion people on this earth rely on herbal medicines.[7] The plant kingdom has provided food and medicine since the beginning of time, and herbs have been used for centuries.

There is little evidence that many popular herbs actually work, and there is plenty of evidence that some of them do harm. Most herbs have the potential for a drug interaction with many prescribed medications. Herbal remedies also have significant side effects. In fact, we strongly advise you not to mix herbs and medications.

Some of the risks of mixing herbs and medications include poisoning, hepatitis, anxiety, tachycardia (rapid heart beat), hypertension, and heart arrhythmias. For example, St. John's wort can cause heart problems when taken with prescribed medications.

Some of the reasons why we generally do not advise you to take herbs are:

- There are limited data on their effectiveness.
- Up to thirty different names may be used for the same compound.
- There is no regulation of the quantity of the herbs you buy, nor are there standards on the correct dose to take.
- There is usually no listing of the active ingredients in the herbs you buy.
- There are insufficient data on interactions with medications or other herbs.
- The side effects of herbs are not well known.

Don't fool yourself by believing that you're not taking medication when you take an herb. Even if it is advertised as being "all natural," if an herb has a drug effect, it will also have a drug-like side effect. We don't mix medications and herbs because the potential for interactions is high.

Part of the intrigue of taking an herb is *not* going to the doctor, but essentially prescribing for yourself. This just isn't safe. Herbs and medications both need to be prescribed and distributed by qualified physicians. Most traditions of herbal healing agree with modern psychiatry that depression is a physical illness. Herbs may be useful for mild depression, but they should never be substituted for psychotherapy nor should they be prescribed while you're taking antidepressants without first seeking guidance from *both* a doctor *and* an herbal medicine specialist.

Our bottom line is that we are not going to "play around with herbs" in pregnancy or in the treatment of postpartum depression.

Homeopathy

Homeopathy is a 200-year-old system of medicine in which disease is treated with diluted solutions of plant extracts. It is not considered safe during pregnancy, and we do not recommend it for the treatment of postpartum depression.

Naturopathy

Naturopathy is a form of treatment based on the belief that disease is the result of blockages in the flow of life force through the body. Treatment is generally acupuncture and homeopathy. We cannot recommend this approach during pregnancy or for the treatment of postpartum depression.

Hypnosis

Hypnosis is helpful if you want to stop addictions, compulsions, or phobias. There is no evidence that it has any appreciable effect on depression.

Acupuncture

Acupuncture has a long history as it has been used in China for more than 2,500 years. It appears to make biological sense for some disorders, but it is doubtful if it can cure depression. We do not recommend acupuncture during pregnancy or for the treatment of postpartum depression.

Communication with Your Treatment Team

Seventy-two percent of patients do not tell their primary doctors they are using an unconventional practice or using a complementary alternative medicine approach—even when they go to their primary doctor for the same condition. Don't be part of this statistic. Don't hide it from your doctor if you wish to use a complementary alternative approach or are already using one.

A growing number of physicians are willing to acknowledge the benefits of complementary support, including yoga, diet, meditation, acupuncture, hypnosis, massage, biofeedback, and relaxation. We support these practices in many instances as we have indicated in this chapter. However, you must be open with your treatment team about your preferences.

One of the things that you must face is that it is easier to take a pill or an herb than it is to do the hard stuff, including diet and exercise. We realize that when you have postpartum depression, you're not going to get up early every morning to go running. However, as you improve and feel better, a healthier style of living will come easier for you. And a healthier lifestyle will help to prevent a recurrence of your depression.

Although we do not believe in the use of herbs during pregnancy or in the treatment of moderate to severe postpartum depression, we are strong advocates of using a full treatment approach and using complementary alternative treatments. Herbal medicine may certainly play a major role in the future in the treatment of postpartum depression. But for the present, stick to what works—prayer, lifestyle modification, stress reduction, exercise, meditation, and dietary changes.

11

Developing a Social Support Network

POINTS TO PONDER IN THIS CHAPTER

- Whenever there's a crisis in your life, you require support from others.
- It is essential that during your pregnancy you build a social support network.
- The most important source of support will come from your husband or partner.
- You need to ask family and friends for their support.
- A doula, a midwife, and your primary care professionals are important resources for support.

Having postpartum depression is a legitimate crisis requiring the same kinds of attention and help as any other health crisis you may experience. Whenever there's a crisis of any magnitude in your life, you need support from others. Pregnancy and childbirth are no exception. In this chapter, we want to convince you of the absolute necessity for building a social support network. You need to make sure that if you have risk factors that make you a likely candidate for developing postpartum depression, that you begin to put together a support system during pregnancy. Finally, we want you to be aware that no matter how courageous

141

and self-reliant you are, if you have postpartum depression, you will need the ongoing support of others in order to recover.

While pregnant with her first baby, LaTasha attended a class to prepare her for childbirth and the care of her baby. She learned about postpartum depression in this class and when she began to see signs of mood swings in herself, she decided she should pay more attention to the support she would need.

"My husband was supportive," LaTasha said, "but I really didn't know how supportive he would be in the delivery room and later at home. So my mother and sister agreed to be there for me during my labor and delivery. I also asked them to spend the first month living at my house so I would have positive people around me all the time." LaTasha had first discussed this with her husband so he wouldn't resent her family and see them as intrusive.

Over the past twenty years, research has shown that social support promotes mental and physical well-being, especially during times of stress.[1] Lack of support, on the other hand, has been linked to psychological distress, and both mental and physical illness.[2] Since the early 1980s, there have been numerous studies investigating the link between postpartum depression and the lack of social support. Nearly every study looking at the risk factors for the prevention and treatment of postpartum depression concludes that social support is critical.[3]

The Component of Social Support

"Social support" refers to connections between one person and another. The smallest social relationship is between two people. However, social relationships can be larger and go beyond individuals to include families, neighborhoods, cities, states, and even nations.

Support refers to help or assistance. This help may be emotional, financial, physical, educational, or practical. The events following any tragedy in the United States, whether a devastating tornado, a deadly hurricane, a rampaging flood, or even a terrorist attack, provide opportunities for social support. People who lose a home, personal belongings, a neighborhood, or a loved one discover that their social support network may suddenly extend greatly. The Red Cross, various other relief agencies, businesses, families, friends, and strangers from all over the country step forward to provide physical, financial, and, above all, emotional support.

In our practices, we regularly see the healing power of social support among women with postpartum depression. For instance, after Rachel gave birth to her first child, her entire extended family took turns staying with her. They cared for Rachel and the baby around the clock for several weeks, alternating shifts in order to help her at this time of crisis because of her postpartum depression. The caring and love of her family aided her recovery.

When Mallory delivered her son, she almost immediately descended into a serious depression. "It took me several months to get better," Mallory says, "but thank God for my husband, my mother-in-law, and my postpartum team. They all stood by me every step of the way and they gave me tremendous support. I could not have gotten better by myself."

We also see too many women with postpartum depression who lack social support, even within their own families. For instance, Cathy, the mother of a new baby boy, recalled feeling all alone once she came home from the hospital. "My parents said they couldn't wait until I had a child," Cathy said bitterly. "But when I came home from the hospital, they didn't come around. In fact, nobody came to see me once I got home with my son. I never felt so alone."

Many women discover that the partner, family, or friends they counted on are not there for them, and many of these women do not have a strong preexisting relationship with a church, work colleagues, or even their physicians.

Husband or Partner Support

The importance of support from your husband or partner* cannot be overemphasized. From the time you become pregnant through the early months of caring for your baby, the support of your partner is invaluable.

The reason for this is that most women regard their husbands as their main source of emotional and physical support. You already know that a significant risk factor for postpartum depression is an unhappy marriage or a relationship that is strained and unsatisfactory. Many studies have found that if you receive support from your husband during pregnancy, labor, delivery, and the postpartum period then you are less likely to become depressed.[4]

This was certainly true for Alisha. "My husband and I have always been very close and loving. We decided when I got pregnant that we would go to classes together and we didn't want anyone else at the hospital during my labor and delivery. We just wanted it to be us."

Alisha adds that her husband, Dave, was a big help at all stages. "He held my hand when I was in the delivery room and that just made me feel his strength and confidence," she says.

Another woman we treated says that neither she nor her partner realized how much help he was until he went back to work just a few days after she was home from the hospital. "When he was there with me and the baby the first four days," Barbara recalls, "he was puttering in the garage and in the basement. He finally told me he was going back to work because he didn't feel like he was being much help to me. However, the day he returned to work, I had a complete emotional meltdown. We both realized then that it wasn't what he did to help so much as it was his presence that made a difference for me."

---

*In this chapter the words "partner," "husband," and "spouse" will be used interchangeably.

While the support of a partner can stave off depression, if you do suffer from postpartum depression, the support you receive at home can have a measurable effect on your treatment.[5] The more partner support you have, the quicker your recovery. It is clear to us that if your spouse is supportive, you will have less stress in your life and your recovery will go more smoothly.

Furthermore, you will be more appreciative of your husband's contribution to the relationship the two of you share when he is supportive. As a result of having a supportive husband, your sense of well-being as a woman, a partner, and a mother will increase markedly.[6]

Suggestions for Husbands and Partners

If you are a man reading this book, you may wonder how you can best participate in your partner's experience in order to prevent or minimize postpartum depression.

These days, you, as a man, are expected to be more involved in childbirth and childcare than your father was. You are an essential part of the pregnancy and childbirth, whereas earlier generations of fathers were not.

During pregnancy, you can play an important role by helping to assess the risks of postpartum depression for your spouse. Furthermore, if you're supportive throughout the pregnancy and she knows you will play a major supportive role during labor and childbirth, the chances of postpartum depression will decrease.

Also, during pregnancy, you can be on the lookout for signs of depression because often there are signals that she could develop postpartum depression. If those warning signs do appear, then you can help her arrange for treatment, either before or after childbirth. Although if you've read previous chapters, then you know that when depression appears the quicker you help her get into treatment, the better for her and your family. It is equally important for you to remember that your partner is an adult who can—even if depressed—participate in decision-making for herself. Don't treat her as a child or as a helpless, dependent individual.

If you see the risks for postpartum depression and you are aware that there is a distinct possibility she may be depressed after giving birth, then you want to make sure not only that you are going to be with her throughout pregnancy, labor, and childbirth, but that you will assist her in developing a larger social support network if the one she has is limited.

During labor, you can arrange to be available to provide support and comfort. By taking a class with her beforehand you will learn how to be most helpful during labor and delivery. However, what she needs most is for you to be positive and encouraging. By talking ahead of time, you and your partner can share your desires and wishes about the way you will handle labor and childbirth. Knowing her wishes, you will be able to be supportive and reassuring while overseeing the birthing process.

During delivery, your role is to be a coach and team player. As such, you will provide encouragement and comfort, which will help to ensure a more successful delivery. Your encouragement and strength will almost always include helping her to feel confident, relaxed, and informed as to what is going on. Let her know that she's up to the challenge and that you're proud of her.

After delivery, your job becomes even more important. Your wife will need you to listen to her feelings and her concerns. And you must do this without criticizing or judging her. If and when she develops postpartum depression, make sure she gets treatment from a postpartum depression treatment team, and make sure you participate in that treatment. Do not dismiss her or trivialize her depression. Remember that this is the woman you love and the mother of your child.

At home, you can rearrange duties and responsibilities so that you take on more household chores as well as be involved in the care of the baby and any other children you may have. And beyond this instrumental help, as a supportive person in her life, keep reassuring her that her illness is temporary and that she will get well.

Depending on the awareness of the family, you may have a role to play in educating the extended family about her illness and the treatment she is receiving. While you're being supportive, try to see to it that other family members understand, become educated about postpartum depression, and are not critical or have overly unrealistic expectations of her. Above all, welcome the help of her parents or yours, if appropriate. Keep in mind that your partner requires at least two uninterrupted nights of sleep each week, even if she is breastfeeding.

When Cathy talked to her husband about feeling isolated and alone, he talked it over with her and immediately called his parents as well as her parents. He told them that Cathy was feeling empty and she needed help. He told them they were needed to pitch in and help. Both sets of parents began calling and visiting within two days—much to the relief of both Cathy and her husband.

Finally, keep talking to your partner about her feelings. Your involvement will be invaluable in her recovery, if she's able to confide in you and share her feelings. Postpartum depression is a disorder that is best approached by you and your partner with openness and a positive attitude. You can give her hope as she recovers.

Support from Family and Friends

Next to your husband, the most important support will come from the people in your immediate family. If you have a close family who loves and accepts you unconditionally (rather than advising you to "snap out of it"), you are among the fortunate.

Remember, a significant stressor during and after pregnancy is feeling alone and unsupported. To counteract this major stressor, you need the help and support of others. While most of us can withstand the stress of one problem or difficulty in our life, it is often overwhelming to have two or three or more stressors at once. Giving birth is a physical and emotional stress, but being alone and feeling as if no one cares how you're doing can become the proverbial straw that broke the camel's back—and lead to depression.

That's where you need your family. Because many of the women we see are strong and self-reliant, they are often reluctant to tell their own mothers and fathers about their postpartum depression. We've also met women who might tell their mothers but not the rest of their families. The "rest of the family" usually means those who are not part of your immediate family or your baby's father's family. We strongly recommend that you tell both sides of the family when you're depressed and help them become educated about this disorder so that they can assist you by becoming part of your support system. Without it, your postpartum depression treatment will be hampered. With it, your recovery can be more quickly achieved. If you absolutely can't bear to tell them you have postpartum depression, start by telling them you have a sleep disorder—and go from there.

Becky, a psychologist, was a very independent and strong-minded woman. She felt she could handle caring for herself and her baby just as she had always handled whatever came along in life. "One day I was just so depressed," Becky says, "that I called my mother and told her how I was feeling. It was hard for me to ask her for help. But once I did it, she started watching the baby so I could get some sleep in the afternoons and I began to feel much better."

Research shows that if you think emotional support is important at this time in your life than it *is* important.[7] You need to communicate your need for support to your extended family and to friends. It's important that you let them know the importance of support at all stages of your pregnancy, labor, delivery, and during the postpartum period. You may need to enlarge your circle of family and friends in order to get all the support you need.

What can you ask your family and friends to do? Here are some suggestions:

- Ask them to just be there for you. If you need others to be there during labor or right after your delivery or when you come home from the hospital, ask them. Let them know that you're not asking for anything else from them—just that they will be there to visit and talk.
- Ask them to help out with things that you're not sure you'll be able to do on your own. This could include helping you to bathe the baby, help with cleaning or laundry, help with caring for your other children, help with shopping or preparing meals, help with reminding you to take your medications, or help with transportation to appointments.
- Don't expect family members and friends to know exactly what you're feeling or how at times you may feel worthless and hopeless. However, you can let them know that if they just offer empathy and compassion that their kind words and warm vibes will do wonders for your recovery.

Suggestions for Family Members and Friends

If you're a family member or a friend, what can you do to help a woman who is at risk for postpartum depression or has developed postpartum depression? Here is a list of suggestions that can help you be a godsend in her getting well quicker:

- Help her develop and mobilize support. She can't and won't do it alone.
- Express your concern. You don't have to have profound words, and you don't have to know how she feels. Just be aware by being there and letting her know your concerns that you will be helping—probably more than you'll ever know.

- Ask how you can help. You may wonder what you can do to help. One sure way of finding out is to ask. She may be unwilling to ask for help, but she may respond when you sincerely ask how you can help.
- Offer hope. To be truly supportive, you must offer hope and reassurance. Let her know that depression is a very treatable illness and she *will* get better.
- Give positive reinforcement. Adults, especially depressed adults, need as much positive reinforcement as do children. When you have a friend or family member who is depressed, you can be sure that frequently her thoughts about herself and her situation are likely to be negative. You will be helping immeasurably by reminding her about her strengths and assets, as well as how much she means to you and others.
- Keep your sense of humor. It's not easy to be supportive to someone who is depressed. However, when the situation becomes tense or the atmosphere becomes very dark, a joke or a humorous way of looking at things can lighten the tension or part the dark clouds—at least temporarily. Don't, however, make light of her depression or make "jokes" about her snapping out of it.
- Encourage healthy behavior and activities. Prior to becoming depressed, many women have been busy and active. However, we know that social activities and exercise can help to ease the symptoms of depression. Encouraging walking, swimming, running, bicycling, and visiting others will be as important as many other aspects of treatment. But suggest, don't tell her what she needs to do. If she can't do it alone, ask if the two of you can be active together.

Support from Midwives and Doulas

Midwives are women who are medically trained and qualified to do vaginal exams, monitor fetal heart tones, and deliver babies—both at home and at a hospital. Doulas, on the other hand, are women experienced and professionally trained to provide continuous support to you and your family during labor and delivery, and in childcare at home. Unlike a midwife, the doula does not perform clinical tasks or provide medical interventions or advice. However, both midwives and doulas can be resources for you.

You already know that having social support during pregnancy and especially during your delivery will assist in the prevention and treatment of postpartum depression.[8] While doula care has only relatively recently been introduced in the United States, the presence of continuous social support during childbirth has been practiced in other countries for centuries.[9] Women in the United States stopped giving birth at home and began going to the hospital in the 1920s. That shift substantially altered the nature of social support provided to women during delivery.

What subsequently happened in hospitals was that female assistants (along with husbands and relatives) were typically excluded, and women generally went through labor and childbirth alone. Medication was often used to calm and comfort women who felt both alone and frightened. It was the natural childbirth movement of the 1960s and 1970s, however, that helped to bring about a recognition of the support women needed. Consequently, husbands were allowed in delivery rooms. The broadening of this support was later extended to doulas, particularly as the benefits of continuous care and social support became more widely appreciated.

Karen Schroeder has been a doula in the Midwest for ten years. "I'm on call 24–7," Karen says about her job. "I'm part of a woman's life." Her goal is to help new mothers be the best mothers they can be by a calm and supportive atmosphere in the delivery room, created by the doula's assistance.

"The problem with our society," Karen says, "is that when women listen to each other, they sometimes only listen to the bad or the negative. What I like to bring to the birthing process is an opportunity for women to find an inner strength to get through the process." For this reason, Karen encourages pregnant women to practice yoga.

A good doula is, according to Karen Schroeder, part of the team during labor and delivery. A doula will promise to be with you, provide continuous care during labor and the birthing process, and stay with you afterward. And a good doula will suggest proper nutrition, exercise, education, and support.

Melinda Cook, a nurse and midwife in Australia, says that moving childbirth from the home to the hospital has resulted in the increasing "medicalization" of childbirth. While this has led to safer deliveries for mothers, Cook says that it is also responsible for the disintegration of a woman's sense of dignity, fulfillment, and autonomy during the birthing process.[10] Additionally, of course, for several decades family support was discouraged in that process.

Recent research related to social support during delivery has confirmed the importance of the support offered by midwives. One recent study found that new mothers who receive "tailored care from a midwife" for a few weeks or months following delivery are up to 40 percent less likely to develop postpartum depression.[11] Another study indicated that a woman who benefits from either a midwife or a doula may chiefly do so because she has a supportive woman to talk with about her experience.

Health Care Professional Support

The social support you receive will, in most instances, come from your husband, family, and friends. Yet your doctor and the nurses who care for you in the hospital can be extremely important in offering you needed support. While the support that comes from physicians and nurses is more likely to be in the form of practical assistance, it can also be emotional as well.

Melinda, after giving birth to her first baby, said that her obstetrician was wonderful. "She seemed to understand how I was feeling and gave me lots of encouragement," she said.

Brenda, during her short stay in the hospital when delivering her twins, was enthusiastic about the care given her by the nursing staff. "They were kind to me during my long labor," Brenda said, "and they checked on me constantly after the delivery. They always anticipated my needs."

Marsha had been sent to the hospital at the beginning of her eighth month of pregnancy by her doctor because she needed bed rest. "I was in the hospital for two months," Marsha says, "and I got to know the nurses very well. I have to say that they were fabulous. They were always there offering me a kind word or encouragement."

If there's one thing that some studies have found lacking in doctor and nursing care, it is that health care professionals do not provide enough guidance in childcare and breast-feeding.[12] In addition, many women who develop postpartum depression feel they were not adequately warned or prepared to deal with depression. However, if you are affiliated with a hospital that offers educational programs for parents-to-be, you should take advantage of them. This is an important aspect of asking for help.

Sue said that she and her husband took every new parent class their hospital offered. "I thought my husband Scott would protest the number of classes I signed us up for," she said, "but he didn't. Instead, we went to all of them and we both felt like we were well prepared for everything that happened from labor through delivery. The classes my hospital provided were terrific."

If you're like many mothers and fathers these days, you may feel ill-prepared to become a parent. However, mother and baby groups that many hospitals offer will help to decrease any sense of inadequacy or even isolation you may feel. Groups and classes will frequently cover such important topics as how to care for your baby, breast-feeding, childcare resources, and parenting an infant.

Hospitals usually have social workers and visiting nurses on staff and these people can be valuable resources when you need someone to talk to or you have questions about any aspect of your health or childcare.

Furthermore, your local public health department may also provide visiting nurse services that can help care for your baby. Additionally, a health department can assist you to find other resources you might need, such as visiting homemaker services and referrals to other family resources.

Postpartum Depression Team Support

When you find a good postpartum depression team to treat you, you should get the kind of medical, psychological, emotional, and parenting support that will augment the support you're getting from your home team and social network.

As we said in Chapters 8 and 9, one aspect of competent treatment from postpartum depression specialists is that they will be there for you when you need them. Your psychiatrist should be available by pager or answering service; we believe that when you have postpartum depression, you may need daily calls from your treating psychiatrist to answer your questions and give you support.

Leslie said she would never have made it without daily calls from her psychiatrist. "I also wouldn't have filled the prescription," Leslie said, "if he hadn't given me a sample card of medication."

Similarly, the psychologist or mental health professional quarterbacking the treatment team should literally be available to you 24 hours a day, seven days a week. Your part in this care network is to use this support to make sure that you get answers to your questions and reassurance whenever you feel overwhelmed or you fear that you'll never get better. We're not suggesting that you call for "telephone therapy," but that you have access to your treatment team if and when you need help.

In the final chapter we will talk about another component of your treatment—being a confident and successful parent.

12

Parent Skills Training

POINTS TO PONDER IN THIS CHAPTER

- Babies are affected almost immediately after birth by care from a depressed mother.
- The negative effect of having a depressed mother can last into later childhood.
- By learning how to interact with your baby you can overcome some of the negative effects of depression.
- Paying attention to both play and discipline can help you send the right messages to your child.

Up to now we have been telling you about the effects of depression on you, with only occasional references to your friends and family. In this chapter, we tell you what happens to your baby when you are depressed for long periods of time.

Researchers have been studying the effects of maternal depression on children since about the mid-1980s. The results of this research are clear and consistent: Children who live with a chronically depressed mother are at risk for many adverse effects.[1] For you, this means that if you fail to receive treatment for your postpartum depression, your baby as well as your older children are very likely to suffer consequences. Therefore, early identification and treatment for your postpartum depression is important for you and your child. The longer your child is exposed to your depression, the more problems he is likely to experience as an infant, a toddler, and preschooler, as well as during the elementary school years.

What Happens to Babies Exposed to Depression

We know the risks for you if you have postpartum depression and go untreated. But what are the risks for your baby? The risks for your baby are considerable. Here are the major risks researchers have found:

Higher stress levels
Abnormal reflexes
Withdrawal
Irritability
Decreased vocalization
Lower activity level
Attachment problems
Depressed emotional expression

When babies of depressed mothers have been studied, it's been found that they often show withdrawal, irritability, low levels of excitability, and flat facial expressions. Furthermore, if you are depressed for as much as the first six months of your infant's life, she is likely to have delayed motor development, emotional difficulties, social problems, and depression.[2]

The consequences of being around a depressed mother begin to appear within the first year of life for many infants. For instance, some babies whose mothers were depressed for the first six months of their life showed growth delays by their first birthday. However, there are less obvious signs that babies are affected by their mother's depressions. Newborn infants of depressed mothers have significantly elevated stress hormone levels (much like their depressed mothers). They also have limited responsivity to facial expressions, show more signs of stress, and exhibit some early signs of neurological delays.[3] Other findings are that babies of depressed mothers have disturbed sleep patterns. They also produce more sad and angry faces and show fewer expressions of interest. They also showed a preference for sad faces and voices.

Four-month-old infants of depressed mothers were more drowsy and fussy, less relaxed and contented.[4] Six- to seven-month-old infants have frequent withdrawal behavior and show fewer positive facial expressions. Furthermore, they display less interest in other people at nine months and, during play, have limited play behavior and seem uninterested in exploratory behavior at twelve months.[5]

Children of Depressed Mothers

Depressed infants grow into depressed toddlers. They then start preschool and have behavior problems, such as aggression. They are sometimes mean to other children and frequently show signs of chronic depression.

Preschool children and toddlers continue to show peer interaction problems, to display anxiety, and to often have behavior problems. Thinking skills seem to suffer, especially for boys, when children live with a depressed mother. And behavior problems continue to increase, with boys, in particular, showing antisocial behavior. Boys are often less mature (than boys who grow up with mothers who are not depressed) and in general less ready to start school.

Why Maternal Depression Affects Children

A major reason for these negative outcomes when children are around you when you are depressed is that your interactions with your child are less social, friendly, and enthusiastic. In other words, when you are seriously depressed, you create a risky environment for your baby. How do you do this?

There are several ways that the home environment becomes more risky for infants and young children. One way is that when you are seriously depressed you are not always able to provide a positive role model for emotional expression. That is, when you're depressed, you're less likely to express positive emotions frequently. Instead, you're more likely to show negative emotions more often. Furthermore, you may not always be as sensitive and as responsive to the needs of your baby as you should be. Babies need lots of face-to-face interactions with plenty of positive attention and a high level of stimulation, which includes the vocal stimulation of baby talk. If you are depressed, your vocal tone is likely to be flat and relatively unexpressive.

If you have serious postpartum depression, the chances are that you will be very withdrawn or intrusive. To be intrusive means that you are sometimes overly involved and too stimulating. Whether you are less involved or overly involved, these reactions seem to be pivotal in determining the effect your depression will have on your child.

Interacting with Your Baby to
Overcome the Effects of Your Depression

If all of the above seems gloomy and like you are destined to harm your baby by virtue of your depression, we have good news. You can override much of the negative effect of your depression on your baby by learning to interact in a different way with your baby.

In our parenting support groups and in individual sessions with mothers and fathers, we teach parents three ways to minimize the effects of depression on their baby. We teach them: (1) To use appropriately stimulating language; (2) To learn to have fun and play with their baby; (3) To learn to massage their baby.

Stimulating language means that you use positive facial expressions when speaking to your child while talking in expressive and stimulating ways. Essentially, this means that you smile frequently, talk often, and interact in ways that make life and the world interesting to your child.

Kerrie rarely spoke to her baby and had difficulty mustering up a smile or enthusiasm when caring for her because of her serious depression. In a parenting support group, she was shown by a charismatic group leader how to talk and interact with her baby. "I didn't have much energy at that time," Kerrie later said. "But when I saw the group leader being so animated with my baby and I saw how quickly and easily she responded, I knew I had to try to imitate the ways of speaking I learned. I found out it wasn't nearly as hard as I thought it would be."

Learning to play and understanding the importance of play is also helpful for you when you're struggling with depression. Although it takes some energy to play, when you learn how truly simple it is and the terrific benefits to your child with basic play strategies, it comes easier.

One of the things that mothers learn and then find amazing is that play actually brings relief from discomfort for babies. Play also teaches an infant how to accomplish tasks. How do they learn to actually grab a ball or a toy? By reaching for it and crawling toward the toy. But, you have to interest your baby in the toy first, place it or hold it away from her, and then encourage her to reach or crawl toward it. It's very simple, but effective in teaching a baby to learn to achieve an end while developing visual-motor coordination skills.

Play, of course, also establishes or re-establishes closeness between you and your baby. Because play is the way babies and children learn, it's a wonderful opportunity for to interact both physically and verbally with your child. While you should be having as much fun as your baby, you are teaching her how to pretend, how to communicate through language and gestures, how to use symbolic thought (symbolic play occurs when one object represents another, such as when a child uses a spoon as a telephone), how to share with another person, and how to abide by rules (such as turn-taking—an important skill for children to learn). Furthermore, your child will begin to learn cause and effect through play. And how can you accomplish all of this?

Here are some tried-and-true ways to play with your baby:

1. Play hand games; by opening and closing your hands, wiggling your fingers, and clapping your hands (while you describe what you're doing), your baby learns to imitate and communicate with you.

2. Sing songs. You can make up songs about almost any activity, or you can use the songs that have seemingly been around forever. These songs include lullabies, alphabet songs, and activity songs ("Here's the way we pick up our toys . . . ").

3. Dance to music. Babies are fascinated by rhythm and movement and will want to imitate you. You can at first dance with your baby in your arms. Later, when he is able to stand and walk a few steps, you can teach him to dance while you're holding his arms.

4. Read a board book. Board books are larger, more sturdy, and very colorful books that babies and toddlers love. It's a terrific beginning to help your child learn as you read aloud and talk about the words and pictures in a book.

5. Take a walk to a park—describe what goes on there. Take a walk anywhere, but whenever you're with your child you should be describing what you see and what's going on around you. When you're driving and your baby is strapped in her car seat, you should keep up an interesting and animated description of what you both can see.

6. Narrate a baby task—talk your way through a diaper change. You can do the same thing with everyday tasks at home—even meals. Describe what you're doing and what you're feeling and how your

baby looks. This stimulates your infant while teaching her about the basics of language.

7. Make a game out of getting dressed. In fact, make a game out of everything. By talking, laughing, and singing, you are stimulating your child and teaching her how to attend to your face and eyes.

8. Have tummy time—get down on your tummies and look at each other. Looking at each other eye-to-eye is great stimulation and your baby will respond to you being on the same level. You can roll on the floor or just reach out to each other.

9. Sit in front of a mirror and make faces at each other. Help your baby learn to recognize her own face while she learns all the fun she can have by making faces. She will learn quickly to imitate you and this is a wonderful way to get a baby smiling and giggling.

10. Roll a ball back and forth. Get down on the floor—often. You can't play with a child by standing above or by being aloof. Instead, get down on the floor and do things, like rolling a ball back and forth. He won't be able to do much more than watch the ball at first, but in a matter of weeks, he'll be able to reach for it and finally to grab it.

Parent Training Groups

We believe in the power of support and training groups for you and your partner while you are being treated for postpartum depression. The primary goal of our groups for parents of infants is to reduce the impact of depression on your child. But here is a list of specific goals we have for you and your baby:

- To create a less risky environment for your baby.
- To increase your ability to be a responsive parent.
- To help you learn the benefits and techniques of infant massage.
- To increase stimulation for your child.

- To teach you how to use speech and language appropriately with your child.
- To teach you new ways to play with your child.

We strongly support infant massage. Learning to massage your baby has some great benefits for both you and your child. For one thing, it helps to develop the bonding process between you and your baby by enhancing a warm, positive relationship, allowing you to look into his eyes and to talk to him as you gently rub his body.

Additionally, massage reduces the stress response for your infant. If you have a baby who is irritable, fussy, or colicky, using infant massage regularly can help to lessen these conditions. Furthermore, massage can reduce pain associated with teething and constipation. If your baby is very active and has difficulty falling asleep, massage can be a godsend as it helps to induce drowsiness and sleep. And then an added advantage is that massaged babies tend to sleep more peacefully.

The final benefit of massage is what it does for you. Being touched and massaged feels good, but it can also feel good when you are the giver. This is an especially important benefit when you are depressed.

Parenting Toddlers

If you have other children at home, chances are that at least one is a toddler. And sometimes it happens that you are still battling depression when your baby becomes a toddler, at about one year of age. Either way, depressed or not, raising a toddler has its own special problems.

It's no accident that the phrase "terrible twos" arose. But your toddler's years don't have to be terrible for you or for her. Instead, they can be terrific, especially if you understand more about toddlers (roughly the span of time between twelve months and thirty-six months).

The toddler years are a time of socialization. That means that your child is learning how to live with other people within the family. He will be learning rules, what's allowed and not allowed, and how best to get along with others. The key word here is "learning." Near the end of the toddler years he will show that he has learned the rules and some of the niceties of society. In the meantime, it is best to be tolerant and patient.

For example, you expect your toddler to learn to share. But it's better to delete the word "share" from your vocabulary until she gets to be about age 3 or 4. It will save you a lot of aggravation if you just change your expectation, or at least delay it for a few months. The same with manners in general. You can begin to teach them, but leave your rigid expectations on the front doorstep.

Since socialization is the process by which toddlers start to learn to conform to social rules, begin to acquire personal values, and start to develop attitudes typical of their culture, it is important for you to do certain things to help this process. Think of these recommendations as discipline and you will have a clearer grasp of how you are to discipline during the toddler stage.

First, it's important to model appropriate behaviors yourself. If you want your child to learn to share, to be polite, or to control his emotions, you must first model these behaviors. Second, in order for your toddler to begin to learn—and follow—the rules you must frequently explain what the limits, rules, and expectations are. Third, you can encourage cooperation by being clear about your expectations, communicating these in a way your child will understand, and having positive consequences when he complies as well as negative consequences when he doesn't.

It's always important with toddlers to find alternative ways to guide and control behavior besides using punishment. Punishment can be overdone and then it loses its effectiveness. However, making games out of discipline, redirection, substitution, and distraction are especially useful techniques to help you deal with an "oppositional" toddler.

The old adage of catch your child being good as often as possible is still good advice. Even difficult and stubborn toddlers engage in many good and loving behaviors. The more praise and attention you use, the better.

Remember that toddlers want to explore and push the limits you set. He is at a stage where he is searching for autonomy and independence while developing a sense of who he is. However, despite saying "No" a lot, he still counts on you to tell him when he's putting himself at risk or breaking rules that are nonnegotiable. As the adult you need to set and enforce limits and expectations clearly and consistently. At times his independence might seem like defiance, but that is only a reflection of his fears and uncertainty. Encourage your toddler's independence and socialization—while still setting limits. You can do this by:

- Being clear in your own mind what boundaries and limits are nonnegotiable.
- Being consistent with that list of nonnegotiable boundaries.
- Telling him why when you have to say "No."
- Letting him choose among activities that are appropriate, but being clear about what are unacceptable choices. For instance, you can say, "No, it's not okay to bite her. That hurts her. You can ask her for a turn or you can play with another toy."

One of the difficulties during the time when you are experiencing postpartum depression is that sometimes you and your husband or partner may not see eye-to-eye when it comes to discipline. To deal with this, you may have to discuss the issue in family therapy or you both may have to attend a parent training group where you have a chance to learn about effective discipline skills.

In our parent training groups, we teach parents that there are three basic discipline strategies: (1) To show warmth, affection, and love to your child; (2) To use discipline techniques to reinforce and increase desired and appropriate behaviors; and (3) To use discipline methods that will decrease and eliminate undesired and inappropriate behaviors.

With these three strategies, you can learn specific discipline methods that help you to follow the broad strategy. For example, discipline techniques to increase desired behavior include giving praise and attention, giving rewards and privileges, using reasoning, and making expectations clear. On the other hand, discipline techniques to decrease undesired behavior include ignoring inappropriate behavior, using verbal reprimands, and using time-outs.

While play, positive interactions, discipline, and guidance all require plenty of energy and patience, you have the ability to do this, even if you are depressed. However, keeping in mind what the alternative is will help you to remember that good parenting is what everything you've done—assessing your postpartum depression risks, getting a comprehensive assessment, and engaging in treatment with a team of postpartum depression specialists—is all about.

Postpartum Depression Resources

Recommended Books for Further Reading

Baby massage: A practical guide to massage and movement for babies and infants, by Peter Walker. New York: St. Martin's Griffin, 1995.

Behind the smile: My journey out of postpartum depression, by Marie Osmond, Marcia Wilkie, and Judith Moore. New York: Warner Books, 2001.

Concise guide to women's health, 2nd ed., by Vivien K. Burt and Victoria C. Hendrick. Washington, DC: American Psychiatric Publishing, Inc., 2001.

Infant massage: A handbook for loving parents, by Vimala McClure. New York: Bantam Books, 2000.

The New York Times *guide to alternative health: A consumers reference,* by Jane E. Brody, Denice Grady, and reporters of the *New York Times.* New York: Times Books, 2001.

This isn't what I expected: Overcoming postpartum depression, by Karen R. Kleiman and Valerie D. Raskin. New York: Bantam Books, 1994.

Women's moods: What every woman must know about hormones, the brain and emotional health, by Deborah Sichel and Jeanne Watson Driscoll. Harlingen, TX: Quill, 1999.

Videos

"Baby Massage: A Video for Loving Parents"
Available at www.iaim.us.com

"14 Steps to Better Breastfeeding"
"Parenting Works! Raising Pre-School Children"

SI Video Sales
P.O. Box 968
Englewood, FL 34295
941-473-2601

"The Happiest Baby on the Block Video"
"Ages and Stages: Knowing What To Do and When"
Available at Amazon.com

"Midwives . . . Lullabies . . . and Mother Earth"
Bullfrog Films
P.O. Box 149
Oley, PA 19547
610-779-8226

"Special Women: How a Labor Assistant Makes Birth Safer,
More Satisfying and Less Expensive"
The Association of Labor Assistants and Childbirth Educators
P.O. Box 382724
Cambridge, MA 02238-2724
617-441-2500
Also available from Cutting Edge Press at
www.childbirth.org/CEP.html

"Ten Things Every Child Needs"
McCormick Tribune Foundation
435 North Michigan Avenue, Suite 770
Chicago, IL 60611
312-222-5022
Also available at Amazon.com

Organizations and Web Sites

American College of Obstetricians and Gynecologists
409 12th Street, SW
Washington, DC 20024
202-484-3321
www.acog.com

Depression After Delivery, Inc.
91 East Somerset Street
Raritan, NJ 08869
800-944-4PPD
www.depressionafterdelivery.com

National Association of Mothers' Centers
64 Division Avenue
Levittown, NY 11710
800-645-3828
www.motherscenter.org

North Carolina Depression After Delivery
behavenet.com/ncdad

Pacific Post Partum Support Society
#104, 1416 Commercial Drive
Vancouver, BC V5L 3X9, Canada
604-255-7999
www.postpartum.org

Postpartum Depression Bulletin Board
rainforest.parentsplace.com/dialog/get/newpostdepression11.html

Post Partum Education for Parents
P.O. Box 6154
Santa Barbara, CA 93160
805-564-3888
www.sbpep.org

The Postpartum Stress Center
http://www.postpartumstress.com/

Postpartum Support International
927 N. Kellogg Avenue
Santa Barbara, CA 93111
805-967-7636
www.postpartum.net

Support for Fathers
www.infotrail.com/dad/html/fathers.html

Notes

Introduction

1. O'Hara, M., Zekoski, E. M., and Phillips, L. (1990). A controlled study of postpartum mood disorders: Comparison of childbearing and non-childbearing women. *Journal of Abnormal Psychology,* 99: 3–15. National Center for Health Statistics (Feb. 12, 2002). Centers for Disease Control and Prevention (2000). Births: Final data for 2000. U.S. Department of Health and Human Services, available at www.hhs.gov/nchs/releases/02news/womenbirths.htm.

2. Desai, H. D., and Jann, M. W. (2000). Major depression in women: A review of the literature. *Journal of the American Pharmacy Association,* 40(4): 525–537.

3. Desai and Jann (2000) and O'Hara et al. (1990).

4. National Center for Health Statistics (Feb. 12, 2002).

Chapter 1

1. Susman, J. L. (1996). Postpartum depressive disorders. *The Journal of Family Practice,* 43(6): 17–23.

2. Burt, V. K., and Hendrick, V. C. (2001). *Concise guide to women's mental health,* 2nd ed. Washington, D.C.: American Psychiatric Publishing, Inc., p. 69. American College of Obstetricians and Gynecologists (Jan. 2002). Answers to common questions about postpartum depression. ACOG press release available at www.acog.org/from_home/publications/press_releases/nr01–08–02.cfm.

3. Gitlin, M. J., and Pasnau, R. O. (1989). Psychiatric syndromes. *American Journal of Psychiatry,* 146: 1413–1422. Kennedy, R. S., and Suttenfield, K. (2001). Postpartum depression. *Medscape Mental Health,* 6(4): 1. Available at www.medscape.com/viewarticle/408688.

4. Altshuler, L. L., Cohen, L. S., Moline, M. L., Kahn, D. A., Carpenter, D., and Docherty, J. P. (2001). The expert consensus guideline series: Treatment of

depression in women. *Postgraduate Medicine,* Special Report (Mar. 2001): 1–107.

5. Hostetter, A. L., and Stowe, Z. N. (2002). *Postpartum mood disorders in psychiatric illness in women: Emerging concepts and treatment* (F. Lewis-Hall, T. S. Williams, J. A. Panetta, and J. M. Herrara, eds.). Washington, D.C.: American Psychiatric Press, pp. 133–156.

6. American Psychiatric Association. (1994). *Diagnostic and statistical manual of mental disorders,* 4th ed. Washington, D.C.: author, p. 386

7. Burt and Hendrick (2001), p. 75.

Chapter 2

1. American College of Obstetricians and Gynecologists (Dec. 12, 2001). Postpartum depression: Will the rates go up or remain hidden? Available at www.acog.org/from_home/publications/press_releases/nr12–12–01.html.

2. Cox, J. L., Chapman, G., Murray, D., and Jones, P. (1996). Validation of the Edinburgh Postnatal Depression Scale (EPDS) in non-postnatal women. *Journal of Affective Disorders,* 39: 185–189.

3. Cox, J. L., Holden, J. M., and Sagovsky, R. (1987). Edinburgh Postnatal Depression Scale. *British Journal of Psychiatry,* 150: 782–786.

4. Georgiopoulos, A. M., Bryan, T. L., Wollan, P., and Yawn, B. P. (2001). Routine screening for postpartum depression. *Journal of Family Practice,* 50(2): 117–122. Wickberg, B., and Hwang, C. P. (1996). The Edinburgh Postnatal Depression Scale: Validation on a Swedish community sample. *Acta Psychiatrica Scandinavica,* 94(3): 181–184.

5. Georgiopoulos et al. (2001). Eberhard-Gran, M., Eskild, A., Tambs, K., Opjordsmoen, S., and Samuelson, S. O. (2001). Review of validation studies of the Edinburgh Postnatal Depression Scale. *Acta Psychiatrica Scandinavica,* 104(4): 243–249. Roy, A., Gang, P., Cole, K., Rutsky, M., Reese, L., and Weisbord, J. A. (1993). Use of the Edinburgh Postnatal Depression Scale in a North American population. *Progress in Neuropsychopharmacology, Biology & Psychiatry,* 17(3): 501–504.

6. Lee, D. T. S., Yip, A. S., Chiu, H. F. K., and Chung, T. K. H. (2000). Screening for postnatal depression using the double-test strategy. *Psychosomatic Medicine,* 62: 258–263.

Chapter 3

1. Freeman, M. P., Smith, K. W., Freeman, S. A., McElroy, S. L., Kmetz, G. E., Wright, R., and Keck, P. E. (2002). The impact of reproductive events on

the course of bipolar disorder in women. *Journal of Clinical Psychiatry,* 63(4): 284–287.

2. Burt, V. K., and Hendrick, V. C. (2001). *Women's mental health,* 2nd ed. Washington, D.C.: American Psychiatric Press, p. 33.

3. Burt, V. K., and Stein, K. (2002). Epidemiology of depression throughout the female life cycle. *Journal of Clinical Psychiatry,* 63(7): 9–15.

4. Wisner, K. L., and Wheeler, S. B. (1994). Prevention of recurrent postpartum major depression. *Hospital Community Psychiatry,* 45(12): 1191–1196. DaCosta, D., Larouche, J., Dritsa, M., and Brender, W. (2000). Psychosocial correlates of prepartum and postpartum depressed mood. *Journal of Affective Disorders,* 59(1): 31–40.

5. Nielsen, F. D., Videbech, P., Hedegaard, M., Dalby, S. J., and Secher, N. J. (2000). Postpartum depression: Identification of women at risk. *British Journal of Obstetrics and Gynaecology,* 107(10): 1210–1217. Bernazzani, O., Saucier, J. F., David, H., and Borgeat, F. (1997). Psychosocial predictors of depressive symptomatology level in postpartum women. *Journal of Affective Disorders,* 46(1): 39–49.

6. Freeman et al. (2002).

7. Connor, Y., and Kendell, R. E. (1982). Prospective study of the psychiatric disorders of childbirth. *British Journal of Psychiatry,* 140: 111–117.

8. Sichel, D., and Driscoll, J. W. (1999). *Women's moods: What every woman must know about hormones, the brain and emotional health.* New York: Quill, p. 121.

9. Sichel and Driscoll (1999), p. 165.

10. Major, B., Cozzarelli, C., Cooper, M. L., Zubek, J., Richards, C., Wilhite, M., and Gramzow, R. H. (2000). Psychological responses of women after first-trimester abortion. *Archives of General Psychiatry,* 57(8): 777–784.

11. Kuijpens, J. L., Vader, H. L., Drexhage, H. A., Wiersinga, W. M., Van Son, M. J., and Pop, V. J. (2001). Thyroid peroxidase antibodies during gestation are a marker for subsequent postpartum depression. *European Journal of Endocrinology,* No. 145(5): 579–584.

12. Priel, B., and Besser, A. (1999). Vulnerability to postpartum depressive symptomatology: Dependency, self-criticism and the moderating role of antenatal attachment. *Journal of Social and Clinical Psychology,* 18(2): 240–253.

13. Chaudron, L. H., Klein, M. H., Remington, P., Palta, M., Allen, C., and Essex, M. J. (2001). Predictors, prodromes and incidence of postpartum depression. *Journal of Psychosomatic Obstetrics and Gynecology,* 22(2): 103–112.

14. Merchant, D. C., Affonson, D. D., and Mayberry, J. J. (1995). Influences of marital relationship and child-care stress on maternal depression symptoms

in the postpartum. *Journal of Psychosomatic Obstetrics and Gynecology*, 16(4): 193–200.

15. Ibid.

16. Buist, A. (1998). Childhood abuse, postpartum depression and parenting difficulties: A literature review of associations. *Australian and New Zealand Journal of Psychiatry*, 2(3): 370–378.

17. Dudley, M., Roy, K., Kelk, N., and Bernard, D. (2001). Psychological correlates of depression in fathers and mothers in the first postnatal year. *Journal of Reproductive and Infant Psychology*, 19(3): 187–202.

18. Cutrona, C. E., and Troutman, B. R. (1986). Social support, infant temperament and parenting self-efficacy: A mediational model of postpartum depression. *Child Development*, 57(6): 1507–1518.

19. Wilson, L. M., Reid, A. J., Midmer, D. K., Biringer, A., Carroll, J. C., and Stewart, D. E. (1996). Antenatal psychosocial risk factors associated with adverse postpartum family outcomes. *Canadian Medical Association Journal*, 154(6): 785–789.

20. Hannah, P., Adams, D., Lee, A., Glover, V., and Sandler, M. (1992). Links between early post-partum mood and post-natal depression. *British Journal of Psychiatry*, 160: 777–780. Campbell, S. B., and Cohn, J. F. (1991). Prevalence and correlates of postpartum depression in first-time mothers. *Journal of Abnormal Psychology*, 100(4): 594–599.

21. Buist, A. (1998). Childhood abuse, postpartum depression and parenting difficulties: A literature review of associations. *Australian and New Zealand Journal of Psychiatry*, 2(3): 479–487.

22. Buist, A., and Jansen, H. (2001). Childhood sexual abuse, parenting and postpartum depression: A 3-year follow-up study. *Child Abuse and Neglect*, 25(7): 909–921. Buist (1998). Wilson et al. (1996). Benedict, M. I., Paine, L. L., Paine, L. A., Brandt, D., and Stallings, R. (1999). The association of childhood sexual abuse with depressive symptoms during pregnancy and selected pregnancy outcomes. *Child Abuse and Neglect*, 23(7): 659–670.

23. O'Hara, M. W. (1986). Social support, life events, and depression during pregnancy and the puerperium. *Archives of General Psychiatry*, 43(6): 569–573.

24. Logsdon, M. C., and Usui, W. (2001). Psychosocial predictors of postpartum depression in diverse groups of women. *Western Journal of Nursing*, 23(6): 563–574.

25. Wilson et al. (1996).

26. Ayers, S. (2001). Assessing stress and coping in pregnancy and postpartum. *Journal of Psychosomatic Obstetrics and Gynecology*, 22(1): 13–27.

27. Brugha, T. S., Sharp, H. M., Cooper, S. A., Weisender, C., Britto, D., Shinkwin, R., Sherrif, T., and Kirwan, P. H. (1998). The Leicester 500 project:

Social support and the development of postnatal depressive symptoms, a prospective cohort study. *Psychological Medicine,* 28(1): 63–79.

28. Gjerdingen, D. K., and Chaloner, K. M. (1994). The relationship of women's postpartum mental health to employment, childbirth and social support. *Journal of Family Practice,* 38(5): 465–472.

29. Logsdon, M. C., Birkimer, J. C., Ratterman, A., Cahill, K., and Cahill, N. (1997). Social support in pregnant and parenting adolescents: Research, critique and recommendations. *Journal of Child and Adolescent Psychiatric Nursing,* 15(2): 75–83.

30. Nielsen et al. (2000).

31. Trotter, C., Wolman, W. L., Hofmeyer, G. J., and Nikodem, V. C. (1992). The effect of social support during labour on postpartum depression. *South African Journal of Psychology,* 22: 134–139.

32. Hofmeyer, G. J., Nikodem, V. C., Wolman, W. L., Chalmers, B. E., and Kramer, T. (1991). Companionship to modify the clinical birth environment: Effects on progress and perceptions of labour and breastfeeding. *British Journal of Obstetrics and Gynaecology,* 98(8): 756–764.

33. Doering, S. G., Entwhistle, D. R., and Quinlan, D. (1980). Modeling the quality of women's birth experience. *Journal of Health and Social Behavior,* 21(1): 12–21.

34. O'Hara, M. (2002). Maternity care coalition: Professional education series. Available at www.momobile.org/conference/2002/Session20Hara.html.

Chapter 5

1. Looker, T., and Gregson, O. (1997). *Managing stress.* London, England: Teach Yourself Books.

2. Mazure, C. M., Keita, G. P., and Blehar, M. C. (2002). Summit on women and depression: Proceedings and recommendations. Washington, D.C.: American Psychological Association. Available at www.apa.org/pi/wpo/women&depression.pdf.

3. Maciejewski, P. K., Prigerson, H. G., and Mazure, C. M. (2001). Sex differences in event-related risk for major depression. *Psychological Medicine,* 31: 593–604.

4. Brown, G. W., and Harris, T. O. (1989). *Life events and illness.* New York: Guilford Press, pp. 385–437.

5. Edwards, D. R., Porter, S. A., and Stein, G. S. (1994). A pilot study of postnatal depression following caesarian section using two retrospective self-rating instruments. *Journal of Psychosomatic Residents,* 38(2): 111–117.

6. Boyce, P. M., and Todd, A. L. (1992). Increased risk of postnatal depression after emergency caesarian section. *Medical Journal of Australia,* 157(3): 172–174. Campbell, S. B., and Cohn, J. F. (1991). Prevalence and correlates of postpartum depression in first-time mothers. *Journal of Abnormal Psychology,* 100(4): 594–599.

7. Hampden-Turner, C. (1981). *Maps of the mind.* New York: Macmillan, p. 84. Ettner, R. (1985). *Risk and culture.* Berkeley, Calif.: Mindbody Press, Chapter 13.

8. Swendson, J. D., and Mazure, C. M. (2000). Life stress as a risk factor for postpartum depression: Current research and methodological issues. *Clinical Psychology: Science and Practice,* 7: 17–31.

9. Ibid.

10. Panzarine, S., Slater, E., and Sharps, P. (1995). Coping, social support and depressive symptoms in adolescent mothers. *Journal of Adolescent Health,* 17(2): 113–119. Warner, R., Appleby, L., Whitton, A., and Faragher, B. (1996). Demographic and obstetric risk factors for postnatal psychiatric morbidity. *British Journal of Psychiatry,* 168(5): 607–611.

11. Callahan, J. L., and Hynan, M. T. (2002). Identifying mothers at risk for postnatal emotional distress: Further evidence for the validity of the perinatal posttraumatic stress disorder questionnaire. *Journal of Perinatology,* 22(6): 448–454.

12. Mazure, C. M. (1998). Life stressors as risk factors in depression. *Clinical Psychology: Science and Practice,* 5: 291–313.

Chapter 6

1. Jamison, K. R. (1999). A world apart. *Newsweek* (Special Issue: Spring/Summer 1999): 79.

2. Sherman, N. (2000). The blues aren't what the doctor ordered: Depression as a risk factor for ignoring medical instructions. *HealthScout,* July 25.

Chapter 8

1. Wisner, K. L., Perel, J. M., Findling, R. L., and Hinnes, R. L. (1997). Nortriptyline and its hydroxymetabolites in breastfeeding mothers and newborns. *Psychopharmacology Bulletin,* 33: 249–251.

2. Llewellyn, A., and Stowe, Z. N. (1998). Psychiatric medications in lactation. *Journal of Clinical Psychiatry,* 59(2): 41–52.

3. Filer, L. J. (1992). A glimpse into the future of infant nutrition. *Pediatric Annual,* 21: 633–639.

4. Ryan, A. S., Lewandowski, G., and Krieger, F. W. (1991). The recent decline in breastfeeding, 1984–1989. *Pediatrics,* 8: 873–874.

5. Winikoff, B., Laukaran, V. H., Myers, D., and Stone, R. (1986). Dynamics of infant feeding: Mothers, professionals, and the institutional context in a large urban hospital. *Pediatrics,* 77: 757–765. Dungy, C. I., Christiansen-Szalaaski, J., Losch, M., and Russell, D. (1992). Effect of discharge samples on breastfeeding. *Pediatrics,* 90: 233–237.

6. Austin, M. P., and Mitchell, P. B. (1998). Use of psychotropic medications in breast-feeding women: Acute and prophylactic treatment. *Australian and New Zealand Journal of Psychiatry,* 32: 778–784.

Chapter 9

1. Ward, E., King, M., Lloyd, M., Bower, P., Sibbald, B., Farrelly, S., Gabbay, M., Tarrier, N., and Addington-Hall, J. (2000). Randomised controlled trial of non-directive counselling, cognitive-behavior therapy and usual GP care for patients with depression. *British Medical Journal,* 321: 1383–1388.

2. O'Hara, M., Stuart, S., Gorman, L. L., and Wenzel, A. (2000). Efficacy of interpersonal psychotherapy for postpartum depression. *Archives of General Psychiatry,* 57: 1039–1045.

3. Salmon, P. (2001). Effects of physical exercise on anxiety, depression and sensitivity to stress: A unifying theory. *Clinical Psychology Review,* 21(1): 33–61.

4. Jacobs, E. A., Copperman, S. M., Jeffe, A., and Kulig, J. (2000). Fetal alcohol syndrome and alcohol related neurodevelopmental disorders. *Pediatrics,* 106: 358–361.

5. Centers for Disease Control. (1995). Alcohol consumption among pregnant and childbearing-aged women—United States, 1991 and 1995. *Morbidity and Mortality Weekly Report,* 46: 346–350.

Chapter 10

1. Jonas, W. (2000). Complementary and alternative medicine: Actions and interventions. Talk at the American College of Obstetricians and Gynecologists Annual Meeting, May 2000, San Francisco.

2. Brody, J. E., and Grady, D. (2001). *The* New York Times *guide to alternative health: A consumer reference.* New York: Times Books.

3. Chambliss, L. R. (2000). Alternative therapies for chronic pelvic pain. Talk at the American College of Obstetricians and Gynecologists Annual Meeting, May 2000, San Francisco.

4. Dossey, L. (1997). *Prayer is good medicine.* New York: HarperCollins.

5. Ibid.

6. Ibid.

7. Tenney, L. (1995). *The encyclopedia of natural remedies.* Pleasant Grove, Utah: Woodland Publishing Co.

Chapter 11

1. Gjerdingen, D., Froberg, D., and Fontaine, P. (1991). The effects of social support on women's health during pregnancy, labor and delivery and the postpartum period. *Family Medicine,* 23(5): 370–375.

2. Skarsater, I., Agren, H., and Denckler, K. (2001). Subjective lack of social support and presence of dependent stressful life events characterize patients suffering from major depression compared with healthy volunteers. *Journal of Psychiatric and Mental Health Nursing,* 8(2): 107–114. Boyce, P., Harris, M., Silove, D., Morgan, A., Wilhelm, K., and Hadzi-Pavlovic, D. (1998). Psychosocial factors associated with depression: A study of socially disadvantaged women with young children. *Journal of Nervous and Mental Disease,* 186(1): 3–11.

3. Gjerdingen et al. (1991).

4. Small, R., Astbury, J., Brown, S., and Lumley, J. (1994). Depression after childbirth: Does social context matter? *Medical Journal of Australia,* 161(8): 473–477. O'Hara, M., Rehm, L., and Campbell, S. (1983). Postpartum depression: A role for social network and life stress variables. *Journal of Nervous and Mental Disease,* 171(6): 336–341.

5. Roy, A. (1997). A case-control study of social risk factors for depression in American patients. *Canadian Journal of Psychiatry,* 42(3): 307–309.

6. Hopkins, J., Campbell, S. B., and Marcus, M. D. (1987). The role of infant-related stressors in postpartum depression. *Journal of Abnormal Psychology,* 96: 237–241.

7. Logsdon, M. C., Birkimer, J. C., and Usui, W. (2000). The link of social support and postpartum depression in African-American women with low incomes. *American Journal of Maternal–Child Nursing,* 25: 262–266.

8. Meyer, B. A., Arnold, J. A., and Pascali-Bonaro, D. (2001). Social support by doulas during labor and the early postpartum period. *Hospital Physician* online journal available at www.turner-white.com, pp. 57–65.

9. Limburg, A., and Smulders, B. (1992). *Women giving birth.* Berkeley, Calif.: Celestial Arts, pp. 3, 4.

10. Cook, M. (1994). The role of social support in midwivery practice and research. *Hunter Valley Midwives Association Journal,* 2(6): 1–3.

11. MacArthur, C., et al. (2002). Midwives can help reduce postpartum depression rates. *The Lancet,* 359: 370–385.

12. Tarkka, M., and Paunonen, M. (1996). Social support provided by nurses to recent mothers on a maternity ward. *Journal of Advanced Nursing,* 23(6): 1202–1206.

Chapter 12

1. Goodman, S. H., and Gotlieb, I. H. (1999). Risk for psychopathology in the children of depressed mothers: A developmental model for understanding mechanisms of transmission. *Psychological Review,* 106: 458–490. Radke-Yarrow, M. (1998). *Children of depressed mothers.* New York: Cambridge University Press. Ashman, S. B., and Dawson, G. (2002). Maternal depression, infant psychobiological development, and risk for depression. In *Children of depressed parents: Mechanisms of risk and implications for treatment* (S. H. Goodman and I. H. Gotlieb, eds.). Washington, D.C.: American Psychological Association Press.

2. Goodman, S. H., and Gotlieb, I. H. (2002). *Children of depressed parents: Mechanisms of risk and implications for treatment.* Washington, D.C.: American Psychological Association Press.

3. Field, T. (1998). Maternal depression effects on infants and early interventions. *Preventive Medicine,* 27: 200–203.

4. Field, T., Sandberg, D., Garcia, R., Vega-Lahr, N., Goldstein, S., and Guy, L. (1985). Pregnancy problems, postpartum depression and early mother-infant interactions. *Developmental Psychology,* 21: 1152–1156.

5. Field (1998).

Index

Dr. Ronald Rosenberg is a renowned expert on postpartum depression, psychiatric medications, and the treatment of depression and related mood disorders in women. On the faculty of Wayne State University School of Medicine, he is both a psychiatrist and an OB/GYN (one of the only doctors with this dual specialty in the entire country). He is a frequent speaker on postpartum depression at hospitals, medical societies, and health-related conferences. He lives in Birmingham, Michigan.

Deborah Greening, Ph.D., is a clinical psychologist who conducts group therapy with couples and families suffering from postpartum depression. She lives in Ferndale, Michigan.

James Windell, M.A., is a family therapist and author of several books including *8 Weeks to a Well-Behaved Child* and *Children Who Say No When You Want Them to Say Yes*. He lives in Troy, Michigan.